Play in Family Therapy

About the Author

Eliana Gil, Ph.D., a licensed Marriage, Family, and Child Counselor who specializes in the treatment of abused children, their families, and adult survivors, is in private practice in Rockville, Maryland. The author of numerous books on child abuse including *The Healing Power of Play: Working with Abused Children*, she serves on the Boards of Directors of both the American Professional Society on the Abuse of Children and the National Resource Center on Child Sexual Abuse.

Play in Family Therapy

ELIANA GIL, Ph.D.

Foreword by
Robert-Jay Green, Ph.D.

The Guilford Press
New York   London

To Cathy, Bill, and Jenny Weber,
who play and laugh heartily with me,
and who like my books because they are
"fat and pretty."

© 1994 The Guilford Press
A Division of Guilford Publications
72 Spring Street, New York, NY 10012

Printed in the United States of America

This book is printed on acid-free paper.

Last digit is print number: 9 8 7 6 5 4 3 2

Library of Congress Cataloging-in-Publication Data
Gil, Eliana
    Play in family therapy / Eliana Gil : foreword by Robert-Jay Green.
    p.   cm.
Includes bibliographical references and index.
ISBN 0-89862-756-7. —ISBN 0-89862-757-5 (pbk.)
1. Family psychotherapy. 2. Play therapy. I. Title.
RC488.5.G525   1994
616.89'156—dc20   93-44074
                                             CIP

Foreword

At a national conference, I presented a workshop entitled "Do Children Hate Family Therapy?" The attendance was good. Too good. Clearly, the title struck a chord because children often seem to dislike family therapy. And who could fault them for it? The fact is that many family therapists either exclude young children or do not know how to involve them actively in family sessions. Thus, in actual practice, the field we call "family therapy" usually consists of treating an individual parent, or only the parental couple, or sometimes an adolescent and one or both parents. It rarely involves young children in conjoint family sessions for any length of time. There seem to be three reasons for this exclusion of young children from family therapy:

1. Many family therapists have not received basic training in clinical work with young children (i.e., child development, child psychopathology, child assessment, or child therapy) and do not know how to relate to children as individuals. In fact, a recent study (Korner & Brown, 1990) showed that nearly one quarter of all family therapists had *no* training in working with children; half felt their training in this area was inadequate; and family therapists who had the least coursework and supervision in child–clinical were the least likely to include children in family sessions. The message is clear—children are often excluded from family sessions because many family therapists are not trained to relate to them.

2. Some of the most influential founders of the field of family therapy (especially Murray Bowen of the National Institute of Mental Health, and later of Georgetown University; the Mental Research Institute [MRI] group in Palo Alto; Salvador Minuchin of the Wiltwyk School and later at the Philadelphia Child Guidance Clinic) were more interested in adult schizophrenia and adolescent delinquency than in disorders of early and middle childhood (Green & Framo, 1981). Hence, these leaders did not focus primarily on developing techniques for the treatment of younger children. In fact, both Bowen and the MRI group believed it was best to exclude children from family sessions (except perhaps for those involving initial observation). They prescribed working individually with the most motivated parent in order to treat the child "indirectly," a view that gained widespread acceptance. It also created a rift between the fields of family therapy and child therapy, which impeded the cross-fertilization of ideas.

3. Although there are some excellent, isolated contributions scattered throughout the literature, nobody has offered a comprehensive and flexible array of techniques for involving young children in the action of family sessions. Much of the family therapy literature in recent years has focused on highly abstract theory—systemic, narrative, and social constructionist models—and has neglected the nitty-gritty concerns of clinical work. Thus, even family therapists who are motivated to include children often do not feel confident about how to do so given the lack of literature, and the variety of ages, presenting problems, and family configurations seen in practice.

This is where Dr. Gil's new book succeeds so wonderfully. By drawing on her extensive training and experience as both a child therapist and a family therapist, she shows us how to use *all* family members' natural capacities for expressive play simultaneously. Never before have we been treated to such a variety of family play techniques that are presented in such vivid clinical detail. Most impressive is Dr. Gil's unparalleled creativity in adapting traditional methods of child therapy (such as puppet interviews and the mutual story-telling technique) to the arena of conjoint family sessions.

Finally, we have an array of practical techniques for use with families of children ages 3–12. Her methods are captivating to read about and described with sufficient depth so that the reader can visualize their application in everyday clinical situations.

For these reasons, I consider *Play in Family Therapy* to be an important publishing event on the topic of conjoint family therapy. This is a book to read and re-read with delight. As such, it belongs in the libraries and minds of every therapist, supervisor, and graduate student who works with children and their parents.

ROBERT-JAY GREEN, Ph.D.
Professor & Coordinator of Family/Child Psychology Training
California School of Professional Psychology
Alameda, California

Preface

During my professional training, I took the usual courses in child development, child psychopathology, assessment and child therapy, and found them inadequate because of their lack of specificity and range. In addition, I found that most of the individuals who taught child therapy classes seemed disrespectful of children and child therapy in general, conveying what I have come to recognize as a general disregard for the field of child therapy by mental health professionals. This minimizing of the importance of child therapy is evident in the low priority placed on child therapy among graduate training programs across the United States. It is only in the last few years that specialized child therapy training centers like the ones at Fairleigh Dickinson University (directed by Dr. Charles Schaefer) and The Center for Child Therapy (directed by Dr. Gary Landreth) have become available. In addition, a National Association for Play Therapy was formed in 1982, which has been responsible for sponsoring an annual conference that gains in attendance each year.

I rigourously pursued child therapy training above and beyond my undergraduate and graduate training by attending workshops and conferences throughout the country. Eventually, I met hundreds of other professionals who shared my enthusiasm for working with children. As a result, I taught several child therapy courses in California and supervised, and consulted with, professionals engaged in child therapy. In the process, I encountered numerous students who initially appeared to be disinterested in child work, or who wondered what possible relevance play therapy could have for work with families.

I also encountered many clinicians who appeared to be uncomfortable with children and therefore did not seek out opportunities to work with children. In fact, many agencies providing internship opportunities have a paucity of child-oriented therapists, or feel inadequate to provide services to young children. Some clinicians, like parents of some of my child clients, question the potential value of "playing with children" and getting paid to do so. Others feel bored or impatient with children who would rather talk to a puppet than to them. And yet with most of the students I discovered that as their level of skill increased (i.e., they knew what to say and do), so did their excitement about working with children. Indeed, direct clinical experience with children is often contagious, and many students who have never worked with children are surprised at how delightful, challenging, and rewarding the work can be.

Family therapists who already have experience working with adults can dip into the vast reservoir of knowledge about the use of play in order to spice up their repertoire of family interventions. It is worth noting that family therapists will find the use of play simultaneously inviting and disarming to family members. Although some resistance might be encountered when attempting to use play with adults, the resistance is greatly reduced when clinicians set a positive tone and convey an expectation that families will be responsive to play techniques and will find them enjoyable and rewarding.

Likewise, those individuals who have devoted themselves to the study of play therapy frequently find themselves in situations in which play work with family members is discouraged, or in which parents are referred to another therapist due to the belief that when therapists see both children and parents, the problem of clients competing for the clinician's time and attention will automatically arise. Some child therapists, who are uncomfortable with family work, may be uncertain about when and how to negotiate individual and conjoint sessions. I wrote this book because I have a deep regard for family systems work and play therapy and believe that the two fields of study are complimentary and mutually reinforcing. I think family therapists and child therapists who have not yet merged their respective theoretical frameworks will be amazed and captivated by the endless opportunities available through the use of play with children and their families.

Acknowledgments

Writing a book is a task that requires concentration, a commitment of time, and an undying interest in the subject matter at hand. Writing is very rewarding when the book is completed, but incredibly frustrating when the book is in progress. It is a solitary task and yet requires that the author be surrounded with a pleasant physical environment, a circle of supportive friends, and family members who are amused and supportive rather than hostile and resentful.

A favorite task in writing a book is expressing public gratitude to those individuals who provide support, nurturance, and intermittent episodes of playing hooky and having fun. I would like to thank my immediate family for being interested and supportive and my close friends for staying in touch by phone, letter, or in person. I would also like to thank the Redwood Center staff in Berkeley, California (especially Ellen Faryna) for their willingness to use family play techniques and report their experiences to me. I am grateful to Karly Kaplan, my efficient and motivated research assistant, who tracked down references, wrote concise summaries, and aptly provided a draft of Chapter 2. Sarah Kennedy, my copy editor at Guilford Press, provided careful editorial assistance, sensitive to the fact that English is my second language. Jodi Creditor, the Production Editor, took great care to develop a product of the highest quality. A book is truly a team effort and I greatly appreciate Guilford's help, direction, and support, as well as my warm professional relationship with Guilford's publisher, Seymour Weingarten.

Finally, I take this opportunity to acknowledge the love, pride, and support of my extended family in Guayaquil, Ecuador, including the families Plaza, Uraga, Valero, Gil, and Arizaga.

Client confidentiality has been rigorously protected when presenting "case illustrations" by altering some combination of the client's age, gender, occupation, or other identifying information. When actual dialogue is presented it is reconstructed from memory using a variety of therapeutic conversations with children, or explicit permission has been obtained to reproduce segments from actual therapy transcripts or from audio- or videotaped sessions. Every effort has been made to avoid violating children's confidences—in addition to parental consent, the informed consent of children was also obtained in those cases in which the children were old enough. Art work is reproduced with parental permission and with camouflaged identifying information.

Contents

Contents

The History of and Rationale for Family Play Therapy

O·N·E

A Historical Perspective on Play Therapy

Child therapy is described by Sours (1980) as follows: "a relationship between the child and the therapist, aimed primarily at symptom resolution and attaining adaptive stability" (p. 275). Child therapy, as a separate and distinct type of work, has been evolving since 1909, when Freud first attempted psychotherapy with the now historic patient Little Hans. The term "child therapy" is often used interchangeably with the term "play therapy," although play was not used directly in the therapy of children until 1919, when Hug-Hellmuth introduced the opinion that play was an essential part of psychoanalysis with children.

Although most child therapists agree that play is the most effective medium for conducting therapy with children, others (Fraiberg, 1965; Sandler, Kennedy, & Tyson, 1980) have raised issues such as whether play produces structural change, and how to define play, since it involves neither dream material nor free association. Schaefer (1993) states, "Play, like love, happiness and other psychological constructs, is easier to recognize than to define" (p. 1). He further contends that "it is somewhat difficult for anyone interested in play and play therapy to gain a clear understanding of what is meant by the term play because no single, comprehensive definition of the term has been developed" (1983, p. 2). However, Schaefer asserts that the potential benefits of play are well documented. In a review of the literature that he conducted, he found such descriptions of play as "pleasurable," "intrinsically complete," "independent from external rewards or other people," "noninstrumental, with no goal," "not occurring in novel or frightening situations" (p. 2). Finally, Schaefer suggests that play is person- rather than object-dominated, and notes that "one of the most firmly established principles of psychology is that play is a process of development for a child" (Schaefer, 1980, p. 95).

Play has also been depicted as a mechanism for developing problem-solving and competence skills (White, 1966); as a process that allows children to mentally digest experiences and situations (Piaget, 1969); as an emotional laboratory, in which the child learns to cope with his/her environment (Erikson, 1963); as a way of talking, in which toys are the child's words, (Ginott, 1961); and as a way of dealing with behaviors and concerns through playing it out (Erikson, 1963). Nickerson (1973) maintains that play activities are the main therapeutic approach for children because play is a natural medium for self-expression, facilitates a child's communication, is conducive to a cathartic release of feelings, can be renewing and constructive, and allows the adult a window through which to observe the child's world. In addition, Nickerson finds that the child who feels at home in a play setting will readily relate to toys, and play out his/her concerns with them. Chethik (1989) makes an important point about the use of play as therapy: "Play in itself will not ordinarily produce changes . . . [hence], the therapist's interventions and utilizations of the play are critical" (p. 49). In addition, the clinician must serve as a participant-observer, rather than a playmate. I would add that play in therapy must be facilitated by an involved clinician in a meaningful way. Some of the most frequent errors made in child therapy are allowing a child to play randomly over an extended period of time, ignoring the child's play, or providing the kind of toys that distract children rather than promote self-expression.

In a recent volume, Schaefer (1993) lists seven common attributes of play behavior: (1) play is characterized by intrinsic versus extrinsic motivation; (2) the child is more concerned about the play activity itself than the outcome or successful completion of the activity; (3) positive feelings accompany play; (4) the child is actively involved and often becomes so engrossed in play as to lose awareness of his/her time and surroundings; (5) play has an "as if" or nonliteral quality; (6) play gives the child freedom to impose novel meanings on objects and events; and (7) play is different from exploratory behavior . . . it tries to answer the question, "What can I do with this object?"

In this volume Schaefer (1993) and his colleagues also explore and attempt to specify the "curative properties of play," that is, they address the fundamental question of how and why play therapy works (p. xi). In doing so, Schaefer conceptualizes a range of therapeutic factors involved in play, including overcoming resistance, communication, mastery, creative thinking, abreaction, role-play (an advanced form of pretend play), fantasy, metaphoric teaching, attachment formation, relationship enhancement, enjoyment, mastering developmental play, and game play. The book then illustrates how these factors are elicited through a variety of distinctive techniques.

As interest in child therapy has grown, and as the number of child-specific referrals has increased, a variation of therapeutic techniques, games, and toys has also evolved. Play therapy has blossomed into a multifaceted and exciting field of study. Early works proposed a range of theoretical frameworks in which therapeutic play was highlighted as an approach or orientation, and recent works have provided practical and precise descriptions of how play might be used with children of different ages, genders, cultures, and who exhibit an array of general and specific problems, or who may be experiencing situational difficulties (e.g., Webb, 1991; Combrinck-Graham, 1989; Friedrich, 1991; Gil, 1991; Haworth, 1990; Martinez & Valdez, 1992; Singer, 1993). These therapists seem to share the qualities of curiosity and a desire to explore, creativity, respect and awe of children's resiliency and uniqueness, sensitivity, and a sense of humor.

THE HISTORICAL DEVELOPMENT
OF PLAY THERAPY*

As mentioned previously, Sigmund Freud was the first to use play in therapy in 1909 in an attempt to uncover his client's unconscious fears and concerns. Hermine Hug-Hellmuth began including play in her treatment of children in 1920, and 10 years later, Melanie Klein and Anna Freud formulated the theory and practice of psychoanalytic play therapy. The play therapy they formulated continues to be one of the most widely respected types of child therapy, and is usually conducted by analysts or psychoanalytic play therapists.

Psychoanalytic Play Therapies

Anna Freud and Melanie Klein wrote extensively about how they incorporated play into their psychoanalytic framework. Whereas Freud advocated using play mainly in order to build a strong positive relationship between child and therapist, Klein proposed using it as a direct substitute for verbalizations. Klein contended that the primary goal of play therapy is "to help children work through difficulties or trauma by helping them gain insight" (quoted in Schaefer & O'Connor, 1983, p. 5). Klein (1937) felt that an analysis of the child's transference relationship with the therapist was the main way to provide insight into the child's underlying conflict.

Freud and Klein took the basic concept of free association, which is one of the basic precepts of adult analysis, and in its place substituted the child's natural tendency to play (Nagera, 1980). Both Freud and Klein proposed the idea that play uncovers the child's unconscious conflicts and desires, and that play is the child's way of free associating. The two differed in that Klein thought the child's play is "fully equivalent" to the adult's

---

* *Note.* This section previously appeared in Gil (1991). Copyright 1991 by The Guilford Press. Adapted by permission.

free associations and "equally available for interpretation," whereas Freud believed that play is not "equivalent" to the adult's free associations, but an ego-mediated mode of behavior, which "yield[s] a substantial body of data," but requires supplementation from a variety of sources, such as parents (Esman, 1983, p. 14).

Psychoanalytic play therapy emphasizes the use of interpretation, recognizing the child's ability to use play symbolically to manifest internal concerns. Further, it is predicated on the analysis of resistance and transference. Nagera (1980) documents that even though significant differences have existed between the theoretical tenets of Freud and Klein from the beginning, the two theories have converged more and more as the years have gone on. Fries (1937), a student of Anna Freud's, emphasized that the two differed in that Freud prefered to withhold interpretation.

Esman (1983) synopsizes the focus of play in psychoanalytic child therapy as follows: "It allows for the communication of wishes, fantasies, and conflicts in ways the child can tolerate affectively and express at the level of his or her cognitive capacities" (p. 19). He goes on to say that the therapist's function is to "observe, attempt to understand, integrate, and ultimately communicate the meanings of the child's play in order to promote the child's understanding of his or her conflict toward the end of more adaptive resolution" (p. 19). The major contribution of psychoanalytic play therapy is the clear delineation of play as a tool that facilitates a child's working-through of internalized difficulties. Play allows the child to bring forward unconscious conflicts and confront his/her affect in a safe way, thereby integrating experiences that left intact could cause symptomatic or acting-out behaviors. Although these thoughts are taken for granted now, psychoanalysts integrated play techniques into therapy slowly, and remained uncertain about how much interpretation was necessary or effective. This controversy regarding interpretation continues to this day, and play therapists hold differing views about how much interpretation clinicians make to children. I use interpretation sparingly, allowing children the opportunity to attribute their own meaning to play, stories, or drawings. Interpretation can often be limiting to children, in that they may have layers of meaning contained in their play, and it is possible that clinicians who offer their interpretations may inadvertently restrict or redirect children's play. If interpretations focus on angry feelings, for example, it is possible that some children may persist in angry expression having elicited the therapist's attention to this specific emotion. Some children may seek to please their therapist, or gain approval, and may easily provide the type of play they believe is of interest to their therapist. I agree with Esman and other psychoanalytic play therapists that clinicians must observe, document, hypothesize, and promote understanding, yet I believe these goals can be achieved without using extensive interpretations of children's play.

Structured Play Therapies

In the late 1930s, a more goal-oriented therapy, known as "structured therapy," was developed. This therapy emerged from a psychoanalytic framework, a belief in the cathartic value of play, and the belief that the therapist should take an active role in determining the course and focus of therapy (Schaefer & O'Connor, 1983). Anna Freud (1945) initially found the use of affective release useful, but based on later experience, she encouraged this type of work only in cases of severe traumatic neuroses. David Levy (1938), stimulated by this principle and Sigmund Freud's concept of "repetition compulsion," introduced the concept of "release therapy" for children who had experienced trauma. What he did was to help the child recreate the traumatic event through play. The goal of reenacting the event over and over through play was to help the child assimilate the negative thoughts and feelings associated with it. Levy cautioned about using this technique before a strong therapeutic relationship had been formed in therapy. In addition, he took care to avoid "flooding," referring to the experience in which the child is overcome by strong emotions and therefore is unable to assimilate them.

Other well-known contributors to the structured therapies include Hambidge and Solomon. Solomon (1938) thought that helping a child to express rage and fear through play, without experiencing the feared negative consequences, would have an abreactive effect. Even more directive than Levy, Hambidge (1955), provided toys to facilitate the expression of the child's recreation of the trauma. He facilitated the child's abreaction by *directly* recreating the event or life situation in play.

Relationship Therapies

Otto Rank and Carl Rogers, who in contrast to the structural therapists were *nondirective* in approach, were the major proponents of relationship therapy. Relationship therapy is based upon a particular theory of personality that "assumes that an individual has within himself not only the ability to solve his own problems but also a growth force that makes mature behavior more satisfying than immature behavior" (Guerney, 1983, p. 23). This type of therapy emphasizes the full acceptance of the child as the child is, as well as the importance of the therapeutic relationship. Moustakas (1966), another prominent leader in the field of child therapy, asserts that the genuineness of the therapist is pivotal to the success of therapy. In addition, he strongly believes that a focus on the here-and-now will result in therapeutic success. Axline (1969) also gives credence to the importance of the therapeutic relationship. Indeed, Axline views it as the "deciding factor" (p. 74). Further, Axline's writings, particularly the widely touted book *Dibbs in Search of Self* (1964), have clearly delineated the benefits and desirability of nondirective therapy.

Behavior Therapies

In the 1960s the behavior therapies were developed based on the principles of learning theory. They include the concepts of positive and negative reinforcement, and modeling, and support the application of these concepts to relieve problematic behavior in children. The behavioral approaches are concerned with the current problematic behaviors, not the past, nor feelings that might have preceded or been contained within the behaviors. No attempts are made to achieve affective release, or any other expression of feelings, or to promote cathartic or abreactive works. Behavioral approaches are applied directly to children in the playroom, or taught to parents for use in the home. This type of therapy has broad application to childhood problems, particularly those that stem from a lack of adult guidance and limit setting. Within this framework, play is used as a means to an end, and is not viewed as inherently valuable in and of itself.

Group Therapy

Early on, several clinicians experimented with putting children together into groups to ascertain the potential for positive therapeutic impact. Schaefer (1980) notes that Slavson experimented with group situations in 1947, guiding latency-aged children through activities, games, and arts and crafts sessions designed to help them "release emotional and physical tensions" (p. 101). In 1950, Schiffer developed what began to be known as "therapeutic play groups," in which children could interact freely with minimal intervention from the clinicians (Rothenberg & Schiffer, 1966). According to Schaefer (1980), what is unique about this type of therapy is that "the child has to learn to share an adult with other children" (p. 101). Group therapy enjoys a certain contemporary popularity, partly because it can be provided at a lower cost, and partly because there has been a growing belief in the effectiveness of this modality. Yalom (1975) documents numerous "curative" benefits provided by group therapy, including: the installation of hope, universality, the imparting of information, the encouragement of altruistic behavior, the corrective recapitulation of the primary family group, the development of socializing techniques, the ability to emulate positive modeling, interpersonal learning, participation in a cohesive group, catharsis, and existential factors such as feelings of self-worth and affiliation. Kraft (1980) maintains that effective group treatment must contain the following elements:

> Leadership, preferably with male and female co-therapists, involves developing cohesiveness, identifying goals for the group, showing the group how to function, keeping the group task-oriented, serving as a model, and representing a value system. In carrying out these tasks, the leader may offer clarification of reality, analysis of transactions, brief educational input, empathic statements acknowledging his own feelings and those of members, and at times delineating the feeling states at hand in the group. (p. 129)

Group therapy continues to be popular as a therapeutic strategy for children and, in some cases, *is* seen as a therapy of choice (Mandell et al., 1990; Johnson, 1993).

Sandtray Therapy

No summary of the major models of child therapy would be complete without making note of the significant contribution made by Dora Kalff (1980), who created sand therapy. Professionals who use sand therapy, which is based on Jungian principles, view the sand tray as symbolic of the child's psyche. Hence, the sand therapist interprets the child's use of miniature objects and his/her placement of these objects in a tray, as well as observes the child's passage through distinctive phases of development. While many child therapists use sandplay in their therapy, it is a distinct theoretical approach, with its own techniques. More recent works on sand therapy, such as *Sandplay Studies* (Bradway et al., 1990), explore the various applications and variations of this model.

Conclusion

A number of theoretical frameworks have been highlighted above, including psychoanalytic, humanistic, behavioral, and

Jungian, respectively. These are the major frameworks therapists rely on when conducting child therapy, and almost every renowned technique can be placed under one of these headings. At this point, it is important to distinguish between the child therapies, and the child therapy techniques. The child therapies are based on a theoretical framework or concept, while the techniques advance those therapeutic frameworks. Some of the child therapies are flexible enough to incorporate a variety of techniques, whereas others restrict the therapeutic techniques. Yet another way to differentiate between the types of therapy employed, would be to separate directive from nondirective styles of play therapy.

TYPES OF PLAY THERAPY

Nondirective, or client-centered play therapy, which the relationship therapists promote, is nonintrusive. It parallels the client-centered approach created by Carl Rogers (1951). Axline is credited with the creation of this specific kind of play therapy, which she delineates in her classic work *Dibbs in Search of Self* (1964). She distinguishes between directive and nondirective play therapy by simply stating, "Play therapy may be directive in form—that is, the therapist may assume responsibility for guidance and interpretation, or it may be nondirective; the therapist may leave responsibility and direction to the child" (p. 9). With the latter type, the child is allowed and encouraged to choose what to play with, and is given the freedom to develop or terminate any particular theme.

Guerney (1983) cites two major features of client-centered therapy. First, it "promot[es] the process of growth and normalization," and second, it includes the idea that the therapist "must rely on the child to direct th[e] process at his or her own rate" (p. 58). The nondirective therapist observes the child's play, often affirming verbally what is seen. In conclusion, Guerney (1983) states, "The realization of selfhood via one's own map is the goal of nondirective play therapy" (p. 21).

The nondirective therapist cultivates hypotheses that are tested over time; interpretations are used sparingly, and, then, only after a great deal of observation. Further, nondirective therapists give the child concentrated attention, and restrain from answering questions or giving directives. Nondirective techniques are always helpful in the diagnostic phase of treatment, and, as Guerney (1983) points out, have been shown to be effective with a wide range of problems.

As alluded to above, the basic difference between the nondirective and directive approaches rests in the clinician's activity in the therapy. The directive therapists structure the session and elicit, stimulate, and intrude upon the child's unconscious, hidden processes, or overt behavior by attempting to challenge the child's defensive mechanisms and encourage or lead the child in directions that are seen as beneficial. In contrast, the nondirective therapists are "controlled, always centered on the child, and attuned to his/her communications, even the subtle ones" (Guerney, 1983, p. 58). Further, the directive therapies are by nature more short-term, symptom-oriented, and less dependent on the therapeutic transference than the nondirective therapies.

The directive therapies are numerous and include, among other approaches, behavior and Gestalt therapies, certain types of board games, filial therapy, and family therapy. Certain specific techniques, such as puppet therapy, story-telling tasks, and some forms of art therapy also lend themselves to being employed in different ways. A nondirective therapist might provide the child with ample opportunities for art work, or to tell stories with puppets, whereas a directive therapist might ask the child to draw specific things, or tell an exact story.

Chasen and White (1989), in their discussion of engaging children in family therapy, eloquently assert the potential value of direct approaches with families:

To the extent that play is involved, families become actively engaged and display high levels of energy. To the extent that it is directed, it is efficient and to the point. To the extent that it is factual, it is directly informative about everyday life. Role playing usually exemplifies all three: It is always involved, it is usually directed, and it is often factual (although it can be imaginative). Particularly notable among its virtues are the enthusiasm with which family members impersonate each other and the honesty with which they represent everyday life as it affects them. (p. 9)

Others have promoted the use of directive therapies in working with children. Martinez and Valdez (1992) suggest that when working with Hispanic children, clinicians take "a more active role" focusing on the child's minority group status as "a central consideration" (p. 85). Their model of working with minority children is described as "therapist facilitated," structured to "access cultural and sociocultural themes" (p. 86), with the overall goal of "empowering the child" (p. 89).

Several play therapists have proposed a rigid separation between the directive and nondirective approaches, and yet I believe that the two approaches are equally useful and can be used in an integrated framework, depending on children's unique needs. Guerney (1983) states a similar point of view:

One need not be only a client-centered therapist to the exclusion of all other approaches. One need not ascribe to the theory of self-growth and self-development from which the approach evolved in order to employ the system successfully. One need only adhere to the approach in a total and systematic way and not indulge in what many practitioners erroneously call eclecticism. Eclecticism really involves by dictionary definition, the bringing together of what is considered the best of two or more approaches into a new integrated whole. (p. 59)

A History of Family Therapy
and Its Use of Play

WITH KARLY KAPLAN

The question of whether or not to provide family treatment was considered a difficult one for therapists of the 1940s. The social work movement that evolved during the era demonstrated the urgency for family focus, but the fields of psychiatry and family work were perceived as separate and kept that way. Available theories conflicted with the social needs of a postwar community, and the psychiatric field faced a therapeutic bind. On the one hand, Freud's psychoanalytic theory proposed that symptomatic behavior was a result of a dysfunctional regulation of the internal structures the id, ego, and superego. Freudians also believed that this deficient monitoring of the self was almost completely separate from social influences, and should be treated as such. As a result, treatment that included the presence of family members was considered detrimental to the patient. At the time, the psychoanalytic technique was so well established that many theorists would not consider other etiologic factors that might explain the emergence and maintenance of problematic behaviors.

As mentioned before, the postwar culture developed an interest in the social contexts of personal dysfunction. This was due, in part, to the fact that traditional psychoanalytic theory failed to provide an understanding of how to respond to the increasing rates of delinquency in children. For instance, traditional psychoanalytic treatment was regarded as slow and tedious in the treatment of schizophrenia. As a result, research conducted during that period on how to treat certain disorders (particularly with schizophrenia and juvenile delinquency) focused on the study of family therapy. In the early 1950s, four groups began to work on the new concept of family treatment. But until a meeting of the American Psychiatric Association in 1956, each group worked without the knowledge of, and in isolation from, the others.

A group later referred to as the "Palo Alto group," which originally consisted of Gregory Bateson, Don Jackson, John Weakland, and Jay Haley (and was later joined by Virginia Satir), began to study the families of schizophrenics (Bateson, Jackson, Haley, & Weakland, 1956). Initially, Bateson and his colleagues elicited information about the family directly from the patient without convening, interviewing, or observing family members (still considered a taboo practice). They documented specific differences in family interaction patterns between the families of schizophrenics and the families of other patients, and became convinced that the link between schizophrenia and family dynamics could be significant.

Two specific differences documented by Bateson's group helped them formulate the notion that a family represents a "system," in which each member is dependent on, and reactionary to, every other. The first difference involved a dysfunctional form of "family homeostasis" (a term coined by Jackson), where if the schizophrenic patient begins to improve, it is likely that someone else in the family will deteriorate. In other words, the family unit is dependent on the schizophrenia to provide equilibrium, and its members are not prepared for the repercussions of therapy. The second problem that the group discovered is the "double-bind phenomenon," a situation in which parents send messages to children that are inconsistent and contradictory. An example of this would be a parent who claims, "I'm not angry," yet raises his/her voice in an angry tone. Schizophrenic children, Bateson hypothesized, avoid parental paradox by speaking irrationally (Bateson et al., 1956).

Across the country, family work was also being done by Murray Bowen, who joined Lyman Wynne at the National Institute of Mental Health. Bowen was an avid proponent of the inclusion of the parents (especially the mother) in residential treatment. His original work at the Menninger Clinic focused on mother–child dyads in the maintenance of schizophrenia. Meanwhile, Wynne had found that individual therapy was often ineffective in the treatment of severe psychoses, and was experimenting with occasional joint therapies.

Coincidentally, while Bowen was conducting his experimentation at Menninger, another family therapy pioneer, Nathan Ackerman, was working there as well. Ackerman was the chief psychiatrist of the Child Guidance Clinic at Menninger, and a psychoanalyst who originally believed in the "keep-the-patient-separate" rule. Through examining his observational research on unemployed miners and their families, he came to realize how important the family element was in shaping dysfunctional behavior. He wrote:

> Among these unemployed miners, there were guilty depressions, hypochondriacal fears, psychosomatic crises, sexual disorders and crippled self-esteem. The configuration for family life was radically altered by the miner's inability to fulfill his habitual role as provider. (1967, p. 126)

As this statement suggests, Ackerman noticed that the roles in the family changed as a result of the fathers "desertion" of the family. This experience and others led him to theorize that family influences should indeed be addressed. He began to occasionally see the family as well as the patient, in his office or in the family's home, as a means of resolving a therapeutic impasse with a difficult child.

Once Ackerman realized the importance of family therapy as a discipline in its own right, he fine-tuned his skills and developed a here-and-now theatrical type therapy approach that led him to become one of the most stimulating and entertaining figures of family therapy. Combining his child and family knowledge, Ackerman realized the importance of *strategic* playfulness in the family therapy session. His theatrical wit, which was often so blunt and challenging that it led his patients into laughter, was seen as an especially quick way to break down defenses. He was skilled at combining a relatively indirect method of rivalry between himself and a family member with the security of half-seriousness, that is, using humor to lower the family's resistance. Ackerman showed that play, when used effectively, produces amazing results (Ackerman, 1970).

Coupled with Ackerman's texts, John Bell's are considered to be the founding texts of family therapy as it is practiced today. Bell, a professor of psychology at Clark University in Massachusetts, stumbled upon family therapy through a misunderstanding. A conversation with John Sutherland at the Tavistock clinic in London led Bell to believe that one of Sutherland's colleagues was seeing the entire family "together" at each session when, in actuality, Sutherland meant that Bowlby had been seeing family members individually, with an occasional family conference (Silverman & Silverman, 1962). The idea of seeing the family together intrigued Bell. He tried it, and in 1958 wrote about its merits in his foreword to Ackerman's book *The Psychodynamics of Family Life* (1958). In 1961, he published his findings in his own work, an essay entitled "Family Group Therapy."

An examination of the theories and practice of family therapy during the 1960s renders a glimpse of what was to come. As theorists were validated by each other and the psychiatric community, they began to develop original styles in their work. Some of the therapies they developed parallel what we now call family play therapy, although it was almost two decades before family play itself was utilized. In 1960, Bateson and his group were struggling to come up with a theory that would explain the interactions that took place amongst family triads. Bateson noticed that schizophrenic families formed dyadic alliances in a random manner, almost as if they were playing a competitive game. Bateson likened these patterns to an unstable five-member game that was described in Von Neumann and Morgenstern's *Theory of Games* (1947). Von Neumann describes a game in which coalition possibilities are constantly fluctuating. Once placed in a "winning" position, a member of the coalition would desert, and find another member to ally with. In therapy, coalitions begin and dissolve in similar ways. Either another member intrudes, or the pair feels so guilty about excluding the third member they dissolve the coalition themselves. Bateson maintains that family bonds are weakened by the constant disruptions of the serious subliminal "game-playing."

Although all of the work described above set the groundwork for family play therapy, its most well-known and influential inventors are Carl Whitaker and Virginia Satir. These two creative therapists included in their early theories two of the most important components of family play: the inclusion of very young family members, and the application of established play therapy techniques.

Virginia Satir, a member of the Palo Alto group, saw a need for a novel approach to enrich the family therapy session. Her 1972 text *Peoplemaking* dealt with this need in two separate instances. Utilizing Duhl and Kantor's technique of "family sculpture," Satir attempted to draw attention away from the diagnosed child and toward the family. She had each member of the family sculpt the others in physical and symbolic relation to themselves. Once the family realized that they were all part of the sculpture, or problem, it became easier to examine resolution.

The other example of a play technique described in *Peoplemaking* was designed to be utilized outside of the office. Satir (1972) suggests that family members aged 3 and above engage in the following:

Seat yourselves in chairs near one another . . . [and] select a way of communicating. For instance, one of you could blame, one could placate, and the third might also blame. . . . Take the physical position that matches your communication and hold the stances for one minute. Then, sit down and play these same communication stances . . . don't be afraid to exaggerate. (p. 82)

Satir then indicates that after 5 minutes of interaction, the players should sit back and take a mental inventory of their thoughts and feelings about the game, namely what meaning the interaction had given the family context. Through utilizing this technique, communication and empathy were found to increase in Satir's groups, and to be implemented in daily activities as well. One of the most interesting features of Satir's method is its emphasis on familial *self*-regulation. In fact, it was a precursor for another type of family therapy called "filial therapy," in which the parent is placed into the "therapist" role (Guerney, 1964).

Twenty years after the development of family therapy, *Peoplemaking* opened the door to a new question: Would other forms of play be as effective as the ones that had been developed? Whitaker, who behaved paradoxically, seemed to think so. His play methods, which he affectionately calls the "therapy of the absurd," consist of spontaneous playful provocations such as appearing bored during sessions or insisting that families not return to therapy. By using these methods he tried to lower the family's resistance, and elicited desired responses such as cooperation and participation in treatment. More relevant to the area of family play, and less sensationalized, is Whitaker's work at the University of Wisconsin, which involved inviting extended family members to sessions. Although Whitaker was not specific about the role of young children in the therapy session at the beginning of his experimentation, he was one of the first to insist that it was necessary. It took Whitaker more than a decade to move from family play therapy theory to practice. Just as the previous pioneers had difficulty proving the validity of family therapy, Whitaker's challenge lay in convincing the psychiatric community that play should be an integral part of the session. In 1981, with a grant from the National Institute of Mental Health, Whitaker and his associate David V. Keith published "Play Therapy: A Paradigm for Work with Families," which attacked the resistance to family play in an ingenious way (Keith & Whitaker, 1981). By providing a list of the similarities between play and family therapy, Keith and Whitaker (both child psychiatrists) managed to address two groups: play therapists who were unaware of the benefits of treating the entire family, and family therapists who were unaware of the versatility of play. Keith and Whitaker were most interested in the "open-ended, nonrational" aspects of psychotherapy, which could be achieved through the use of play. In addition, since they proposed that their goal in family therapy was to "have an experience with the family," they found play enhanced the opportunity for a mutual experience (p. 244). The article eloquently describes why children are such an important part of the healing process:

> Modern child psychiatry worries about children in family therapy being overlooked and excluded. . . . It is important to include children because of their developmental needs. . . . Families need the presence of children in therapy to stay alive. We find again and again that families change less and more slowly when children are not part of the therapy process. (Keith & Whitaker, 1981, p. 244)

The article also vividly outlines the potential uses of play:

> Whole scenes of child horror or child aggression can be acted out on the blackboard, with paints or with crayons. The maneuvers of a huge army can be played out on the floor. Schools, hospitals, cities, countries, mothers and fathers, therapists, children can all be bombed. All of these things have a quality of tremendous power because of their isolation and their ultimate far-out quality. They are not merely civilized representatives of everyday living, they are extrapolations to the grossest, crudest, most distorted exam-

ples or figures. In a way, the play therapy room is like modern movies, with science fiction, sexual abnormality, murder, suicide and sadism. All this is freely available and experienced nonchalantly, thus freeing the child to be more comfortable with his own crazy, infantile, exotic inner self. His internal primary experience is opened up to the interpersonal world. (p. 245)

Although Keith and Whitaker did not give many specific descriptions of the play they used with families, their general guidelines for therapists included sitting on the floor; holding children on the lap; exchanging roles and talking "through" people; de-triangulating family members; laughing with and at them; teaching them to act out through paradoxical interventions, such as asking one member to help another engage in the same behavior he/she is; talking silly; making jokes; acting more delusional than a client; acting on impulse even if the behavior seems absurd; and switching generations, for example, feigning crying if a child refuses to play.

Keith and Whitaker stated they were "always prepared to begin to play in therapy" (p. 251), that is, they routinely asked parents to bring their children and had toys available. However, they listed several situations in which play seemed particularly relevant, including when the therapist feels defeated, when there is a long-standing pathology, when the family has no sense of itself, when there is generational confusion with an abnormally "parentified" child, when confronted with a schizophrenic impasse, when the family declares itself normal, when there is cultural/social class dissonance, when the therapist is excluded, and when the family is "crazy and dedicated to chaos" (p. 252). They further stated that play is less effective with very rigid families, when there has been a death in the family or any other "sacred" situation, when the therapist is too anxious to play or gets carried away with playfulness, or when the play is designed exclusively to decrease the family's anxiety, since they found that anxiety is required to provide a momentum for change.

As the reader will recall, the issue of how much time therapy takes arose earlier. Indeed, family therapy itself had been an answer to the slow, tedious treatment of schizophrenia. Play therapy, in turn, now seemed to be an answer to the slow and tedious family therapy practiced before Keith and Whitaker came along. In this way, play therapy became a link in the search for a better theoretical mousetrap—a better idea for those family therapists who were as comfortable with experimentation as Whitaker and Satir.

Other family therapists were not as prepared to deal with the foreign world of family–play combinations. The 1970s had only a scattering of references on this topic (e.g., Bloch, 1976; Dowling & Jones, 1978; Villeneuve, 1970; and Zilbach, Bergel, & Gass, 1972). It may be that family play was seen as a passing fad and not given the recognition it needed to advance. In comparison to family therapy, it was founded on a much smaller scale, and the idea of it elicited much less interest. It is also possible that many family therapists felt that play was too complex or too abstract to be used in a practical manner in family sessions, or that the techniques involved were difficult to teach. For example, Kobak and Waters (1984) wrote "It is as difficult to write about play and how to interact playfully as it is to give someone lessons in being funny" (p. 96). In addition, the fact that family play techniques were proposed and demonstrated by such charismatic and exceptional therapists might have also had the paradoxical effect of making the very techniques they demonstrated with ease seem impossibly prohibitive to the standard clinician. Chasin and White (1989) state that "in fact, in actual practice, children are more frequently excluded than included in family therapy" (p. 5), and go on to cite that children are omitted from family sessions for the following reasons: to "protect them from information or actions that might harm them" (p. 6); due to clinician's theoretical orientations that insist on adult work exclusively; because clinicians believe that "the ultimate key to the solution lies in the parental subsystem" (p. 6); because seeing the family alone is the most "efficient way to help the family" (p. 6); because clinicians fear that working with adults and children is impossible because bored children will distract families from the important work of therapy or, alternately, working with children using play techniques might alienate the family. Lastly, Chasin and White write that "some therapists are experienced and confident working with children and with adults, but not in the same session. They may resist including both because the techniques they use with adults and with children have so little common ground" (p. 6). These authors propose several techniques (primarily role-playing and active engagement) which effectively achieve a common ground.

In 1985 Ariel, Carel, and Tyano made a significant contribution to the use of play with families by urging the use of make-believe play, which they believe to be a "singularly rich and flexible medium of expression and communication" (p. 10). They suggest that therapists who engage the family in make-believe games heighten their choices of direct and indirect channels of communication. Instead of talking out their transactions, the family who uses make-believe play, enacts or plays them out. More importantly, Ariel et al. clearly encourage the active and meaningful participation of young children in the therapeutic session. They also point to the paradoxical nature of make-believe play in which someone is pretending to do something, say something, or be someone else. They encourage the therapist to take positions vis-à-vis the family's make-believe play, including being an audience, director, or actor; or assuming a variety of other roles such as observer, commentator, interpreter, critic, planner, organizer, designer, or generator of ideas. The authors conclude that using make-believe play allows the therapist to learn about the family's emotional life, wishes and aspirations, strengths and weaknesses, and potentialities.

Kobak and Waters (1984) note that play can be viewed as a metacommunication and as such "allows activities to occur in a novel setting, in which they do not result in their usual consequences" (p. 95). Based on studies of animal play, they maintain that play in family sessions can be responsive to a variety of manipulations, which can assist the family to find new opportunities for change. This is accomplished primarily by "the therapist's repetitive insistence on experimental behavior: starting and stopping sequences, making enactments, reordering, interrupting and reframing interactions, exaggerating or ignoring particular items of data" (p. 96). In encouraging these manipulations, therapists are insisting on experimental behaviors in the hopes of transforming old issues and patterns into something new and different. They call these strategies "liminal play," which involves some mixture of planned direction and an open agenda. Kobak and Waters caution that these techniques require risk taking on the part of the therapist, and that more than a technique, liminal play is "a spirit, mood, and metacommunication" (p. 96).

Joan Zilbach (1986) did a masterful job of tracing the history of play within family therapy formats. (A recent book by Schaefer and Carey (1994), compiles many of the significant articles which advanced and supported the possibility of using play in family therapy.) Zilbach cites Ackerman (the father of family therapy) and Satir (the mother of family therapy) as rigorous advocates of the inclusion of children in almost all of the family sessions, including young children. Zilbach notes that although Satir discussed the inclusion of children in the initial interview with families in *Conjoint Family Therapy* (1964), and emphasized verbal techniques with children, and other techniques such as movement, dance, games and drama, Satir did not include a discussion of play in family therapy.

Zilbach notes that Minuchin always included children in his consideration of the family structure and took particular notice of young children within the family. She contends that, once again, play is not explicitly described, although it is encouraged, in many of his writings. He mentions the use of play materials, such as small chairs and quiet toys, and play techniques are included in many of his clinical vignettes (Zilbach, 1986). For example, when meeting with a family of three children under the age of 6, Minuchin relates that the "therapists, parents, and children sat on the floor building towers and racing cars" (p. 32). Zilbach notes: "Bits and pieces of play are occasionally included within other structural case descriptions of families. However, they are dificult to find, incomplete, and not marked by any special attention" (1986, p. 33).

Zilbach describes Whitaker as "an openly playful therapist," "an enthusiast and one of our few strong allies in regard to children and play" who is emphatic about the importance of play with children and families (p. 34). Zilbach goes on to say that Whitaker had particular types of play that he enjoyed with families, which might not be easy to incorporate for other family therapists. In particular, he developed a technique called "play-battling," which includes some aggressive and intrusive play with children. Whitaker described an example of this technique: "If they bite, we bite back or push their arms into their mouths. We talk silly and expand their sadistic fantasies of tearing heads off, poking eyes, or knocking brains out" (Keith & Whitaker, 1977, p. 120). Whitaker claimed that this kind of rigorous play often becomes a vehicle through which unconscious material will surface in dreams or in artwork.

Some therapists such as Fulweiler (Haley & Hoffman, 1967) encouraged the young child's participation in parent–child conjoint sessions once the child was "old enough to participate," yet offered few guidelines as to how that determination should be made (p. 20). Most family therapists use subjective criteria such as when the child can engage in verbal interaction, or when the therapist feels comfortable with the child. Fulweiler may, in fact, represent a majority view, with his reliance on a family systems theory to explain his exclusion of young children. He believed that therapy sessions are most useful with triads (two parents and one child combinations) because with more than three people the number of interactions far exceed the clinician's ability to observe and respond.

Zilbach also mentions Montalvo and Haley's article "In Defense of Child Therapy" (1973), in which there is an extensive discussion of the problem of excluding children from family therapy, and advice to family therapists that they consider including play, since it could be used to enhance positive changes in the child as well as the family. Guttman (1975) and Villeneuve (1979) also discuss the importance of child participation, and the lack of documentation and description of methods for involving children, emphasizing the necessity for concrete, action-promoting modes of expression.

Family play therapy never gained the momentum it could have during the 1960s and 1970s, and this book speculates on some of the reasons. This is the case even though several noteworthy efforts, in addition to those mentioned above, were made throughout these decades. Irwin and Malloy (1975) reviewed family assessment techniques when writing their article on family puppet interviews, noting that "family therapists have explored numerous innovative techniques for facilitating meaningful communication and interaction among family members" (p. 170). These techniques include a Family Rorschach; filial therapy; conjoint family sessions; asking family members to plan something to do together; assigning family tasks, family art work; instructing families to arrange each other into relational tableaus; and asking families to develop family collages, murals, and paintings. Several board games have been designed for families to play together. *The Changing Family Game* (Berg, 1982) helps children cope with divorce, and *Solutions* (Blechman, Kotanchik, & Taylor, 1981) and *The Family Contract Game* (Blechman, 1974) help families improve their problem-solving skills. Irwin and Malloy (1975) report on the usefulness of interviewing families using puppet therapy (see Chapter 4). In addition, some play techniques have been implemented in group therapy (Hoffman & Rogers, 1991). Irwin and Malloy (1975) state that all these activities "share a common purpose: namely to stimulate verbal and nonverbal communication, revealing how a family mobilizes itself toward a goal or task" (p. 181). Although these creative interventions have been documented, and may be used sporadically by clinicians, techniques that employ the use of play with families have never become widely accepted or employed by either family therapists or play therapists. The literature on children in family therapy has been sparse at best, and when therapy of children is discussed, it is with older children and adolescents, who are often more resistant to play techniques individually or in family sessions.

In addition to some of the earliest proponents of the use of play with families discussed earlier, Combrinck-Graham (1988), Zilbach (1986), Scharff and Scharff (1987), and, more recently, Ariel (1992) have also upheld the idea of including children in family therapy sessions and engaging families through the use of play techniques. Combrinck-Graham states that children often bring an important, not previously encountered, viewpoint to therapy, and suggests that play allows them to reveal their true feelings in comfort. She notes that in everyday contexts children and adults share "very little common ground" (p. 6), and that the therapist must help families achieve balance between child- and adult-centered activities. Combrinck-Graham has found it useful to encourage families to do kinetic family drawings; engage in free play or free-form coloring; and role-play different situations, by having, for example, family members impersonate each other. She finds that these activities encourage family members to acquire mutual empathy.

Zilbach believes that play is not taken seriously because adults do not understand that play is children's "work." In contrast, she finds that play allows for the direct expression and enactment of important family material; reduces the anxiety of adults as children become absorbed in a repetitive and engrossing activity; and allows children to contain their own anxiety. Zilbach finds that children in family sessions will quickly reveal the family's primary concern (e.g., when a child draws a storm as parents quarrel): They can also serve as allies and cotherapists by helping the rest of the family overcome their resistance to attending therapy, and as the early detectors of underlying problems. This therapist suggests the use of simple play materials such as paper, magic markers, crayons, Playdough, baby dolls, and family figurines. She suggests that "a particular kind of toy may be introduced for a specific purpose. For example, the nonverbal, playful release of aggression is facilitated by having an object that is designated for hitting . . . a large, indestructible pillow, or . . . a plastic 'Sock-O' which moves from side to side as it is punched" (p. 136).

Scharff and Scharff find that young children who understand less about family defenses often "blurt out" important facts without there being any retaliation from other family members. Further, observing how family members react to children's behavior is often a good barometer of general family dynamics. These therapists advocate the utilization of several strategies in family sessions with young children, including the use of play materials; allowing children to play while other family members talk; and the use of cotherapists who are primarily responsible to the child and/or family. These suggestions do not include play as a tool for adults as well as children. Scharff and Scharff also recommend linking the child's play behavior with the therapy being conducted with the family: For example, clinicians can ask a child to elaborate on his/her drawings or play; they can use the child's elaboration as a metaphor for family interaction; or a direct link may be made such as "Johnny seems to be drawing the family's problem." They caution that this direct technique may feel threatening or intrusive to young children, and thus may be more effective with older children. As described by Scharff and Scharff, play in family sessions can be central when the focus is on the child, or more or less designed to decrease anxiety and assess family responses when children are allowed to play while other family members talk.

There has been some deliberation regarding the use of conjoint play therapy for children and their parents. Safer (1965) describes conjoint play therapy as a variation of family treatment, in which the goal is to limit conflictive interaction between the child and his/her parents. The therapy occurs in a traditional playroom setting and the child selects play activities in which the parents participate. The goals of conjoint play sessions are to allow the clinician opportunities to examine typical interactive patterns and offer alternatives to detrimental behaviors. The clinician, who remains primarily child-centered while observing the child's play, interprets it in the context of the family. In other words, the play "represents and mirrors" the dysfunctional parent–child relationship.

Griff (1983) developed "Family Play Therapy," a short-term technique used with children and families at the therapist's discretion as an adjunct to other kinds of intervention techniques. Griff states:

> Family play therapy provides an approach wherein parents can learn more effective parenting skills and styles of interaction in an environment that not only facilitates their receptiveness to this information, but also provides a medium that is comfortable for their children. This technique allows the therapist to be a role model for parents who previously had been exposed to deficient role models. It also provides a controlled and nonthreatening environment in which parents can comfortably experiment with change. (p. 67)

Griff describes the use of his technique as flexible—that is, it can be utilized at any point during treatment after a relationship of mutual trust exists between the therapist and family. The technique consists of contracting for about eight to ten family therapy sessions; choosing one or two specific goals; breaking the goals down into smaller, attainable steps; asking parents and children to list their favorite games or play activities; matching activities to the play style of the family; introducing and leading the activities; modeling new patterns and skills; and encouraging parents and/or children to initiate and implement their new skills independent of the sessions. Griff explains that "[Family play therapy] does not commit one to a specific technique that may or may not match a particular family. . . . Inherent in this model is a flexibility in use, location, and mode: short-term and flexible and designed to remove families from their recurring cycles of failure and fear concerning change itself" (p. 75).

Conway (1971) offered conjoint family therapy to ten families containing a first- or second-grade child who had a low "classroom adjustment" relative to his/her peers. She found that families receiving conjoint family sessions significantly decreased their amount of negative interactions and significantly increased their ratio of positive to negative interactions. This study did not employ play strategies; rather, other techniques were used to facilitate the affective communication of family members. Sheedy (1978), using a small sample of four families who received conjoint family sessions that included play techniques found that adult participants experienced the sessions as "out of the ordinary; an evocative and emotional experience which elicits thoughts and feelings which run the gamut of the human experience" (p. 3907-B).

Ariel (1992) has made a significant contribution to our understanding of play, by developing a method of analyzing children's pretend and make-believe activities. Ariel found himself concerned that play "seemed to defy scientific description and explanation," and felt it could profit considerably from "the standards of rigor and precision" practiced in the disciplines of linguistics, semiotics, logic, and human ethology, which he had studied (p. xi). As a result, Ariel has spent the last 15 years of his life researching and developing his theoretical and practical knowledge of the types of play mentioned above, in order to expand current knowledge in these areas. Play, he observes, was like "a new continent that had been discovered, yet not fully explored" (p. xii).

There has been great pioneering work by family therapists and play therapists alike advocating for the inclusion of children in family sessions, the use of play techniques to actively engage children in the sessions, and the development of creative and energetic techniques that might give adults and children a common ground by which to communicate and resolve their conflicts. At the same time, there have been minimal research efforts that document the ways in which play techniques might be useful techniques in working with children and their families, and research efforts must be undertaken to study the effectiveness of conjoint family sessions with young children in which play is introduced as a family technique. The following chapters will draw on available resources, and offer a rationale for the use of play within family therapy sessions.

T·H·R·E·E

A Rationale for Integrating Play Therapy with Family Therapy

The integration of play with family therapy strengthens both therapeutic approaches. As described in Chapter 1, play therapy offers children an opportunity to release pent-up emotions; express themselves verbally, nonverbally, and through their use of symbols; compensate for problems in reality; find solutions to problems; and rehearse the myriad situations children might encounter through pretend play. The goal of play therapy is to assist children to identify and express their feelings in healthier, nonsymptomatic ways, as well as to encourage the working through of difficult emotions while finding and using alternative nonproblematic behaviors.

Family therapy focuses on the interplay between family members who collectively form a whole, or system, that can experience a wide range of functional difficulties. As discussed in Chapter 2, although family systems often include young children, family therapists have been reluctant to include young children in family therapy sessions. The earliest clinical task of family therapy is to assess the family's functioning, and identify problems, solutions the family has attempted, symptom origins, the purpose and maintenance of problems, as well as interactional patterns that create or support the symptomatic behaviors and impede the resolution of conflicts. Although most clinicians choose to interview adults and adolescents in an effort to gauge important verbal and nonverbal information, they often ignore young children by situating them far away in family meetings and giving them something to "keep them busy" while the important therapy work takes place. And yet young children may often be in the best position to alert clinicians to the family's underlying concerns: They do not usually have a vested interest in conscious or unconscious disguises and they have a keen ability to witness or sense family problems. Further, children can communicate on many more dimensions than adults, hence clinicians can benefit greatly from observing, listening, and decoding their myriad communications.

Family therapists and play therapists share a noble trait: They are by far the most creative and dynamic therapists in existence. Family therapists, in particular, have designed and enhanced the use of a host of expressive techniques, including movement, role-play, psychodrama, family sculpting, as well as others that engage the family's participation in a dynamic way, either by intensifying or replacing verbal communication. It is mystifying, therefore, that family therapists (with the brilliant exceptions mentioned in earlier chapters) have been timid to create, use, or champion more opportunities to engage young children in family treatment. This reluctance may illuminate a general reluctance to view children as interesting or gifted communicators, particularly when their ability to use language is not fully developed. What most therapists do with young children, instead, is attempt to impose the adult's world on them. When this fails, and it usually does with children who cannot interact verbally, clinicians relegate them to obscure positions in therapy sessions, in which they are only worthy of attention when parents complain about their behavior or consult about how to deal with general behavioral problems. Even then, clinicians may choose to overlook the obvious benefits of observing parent–child interactions, and may meet with the parents alone. This chain of events occurs in spite of the fact that

Keith and Whitaker (1981), as well as others, caution that "families change less and more slowly when children are not part of the therapy process" (p. 244).

Revealing a similar pattern, play therapists are most comfortable with children and child therapies, and often find adults, particularly a group of adults, intimidating and overwhelming. These therapists tend to avoid making contact with older family members, save for the necessary intake, progress reports, and termination meetings.

CHILDREN'S AND ADULTS' SPHERES OF FUNCTIONING

Children do not rely exclusively on language. Early on, their language is rudimentary, hence they cannot and do not rely on verbal expression. The toddler who points, squinches his face, clenches his fists, and bangs his bed repeating the word "ba-ba" is a master communicator, who by using both verbal and nonverbal communication gets his point across. Children rely on and use facial expressions, intonations of voice, physical movements, and postures to communicate, whereas adults rely primarily on verbal communication, a far more limited repertoire.

When adults limit themselves to demanding and responding only to verbal cues from children, they are imposing the adult world on them. This imposition is unfortunate and unnecessary—a wasted opportunity for ample and enjoyable contact with children. Children are dependent on others for their very survival and their needs are often misunderstood or overlooked when adults limit the ways in which they listen. Children's behaviors must be decoded. Hence, it is wise parents and clinicians who play detective, who always ask themselves what certain behaviors and/or play scenarios mean, as opposed to making rigid or thoughtless interpretations of children's behavior. Adults who view children's tears rigidly as indicating "sadness" may be unable to understand a child who cries tears of joy or fatigue. Hence, when rigid interpretations are made, parents may comfort and reassure children who instead may need a nap, or a good hearty laugh.

Young children are inherent explorers, taking in the environment with a hungry interest. They are sensuous beings, who initially obtain information through touching, tasting, smelling, and hearing. Touch, in particular, seems to supply children with endless information as they grab, push, pull, and savor things around them. When adults curtail, withdraw, punish, and redirect children's exploration, in an effort to maintain order or control, they impose their world on children. Children are therefore deprived of the vast richness of their exploration, and restricted to those things adults direct them to explore, which represents a much more limited realm of experience.

Children have the gift of fantasy, which unfortunately decreases over time. They can turn a simple chair into a fortress, a car, a train, a house, a horse to ride, and countless other things. Sadly, adults lose this ability as they mature. Often, adults do not know how to play with children, who pour imaginary tea in saucers and insist that adults tell them if the tea needs sugar or if it is just right. To their own detriment, adults (including clinicians) may play reluctantly with children, unable to utilize their once ample imagination. When they play in a disengaged or rote manner, they miss entering the richness of children's worlds. When adults are able to relate to children and enter their worlds, a dimension of contact is achieved which solidifies mutual relatedness or emotional connectedness. Because parents and therapists alike are too frequently unavailable to children on this deeper level of contact, the adult world tends to triumph. Children end up playing in a solitary fashion, comfortable and yet disengaged.

Children make full use of their experiences by creating fantasies and stories. Who can doubt that a child who tells a story about a prince slaying a dragon is speaking metaphorically about his/her own drive toward mastery, his/her own desire to overcome fear and danger? Sadly, adults forget how to use metaphors to educate children, and to respond to and address children's concerns in a useful way. Adults are often stymied when asked to make up a story, and may become dependent on books they read over and over, which children enjoy nevertheless. Adults keep doors unopened when they do not rediscover skills they discarded in favor of the adult world of rational living.

These failures to make contact with children can create numerous parent–child difficulties, such as occur when unresponsive or withdrawn parents let their children play in an isolated fashion because the parents feel incompetent or inadequate when playing with them; or occur when parents remain baffled about their children's needs, or how to reassure them, because they view their behavior in a linear fashion, or fail to decode the full range of children's communications. Parents may also become resentful because they experience unrewarding exchanges with their children, and as a result avoid them. Parents may even become intrusive in an effort to understand children's play through interrupting and asking too much, rather than watching for the hidden meanings and symbols of the play. All these factors that stem from a lack of understanding about children's development and communication styles can lead to disharmony, resentments, distancing and conflict, and overall lack of meaningful contact, which can be avoided by entering and enjoying children's worlds.

Unfortunately, parents are not the only ones who can experience these limitations; therapists do too! When children are brought to clinicians for a multitude of problems and concerns, clinicians often fall into the same trap as parents do by limiting their horizons and contact with the children, and by imposing expectations and behaviors on them that offer few opportunities for growth. My basic contention is that adults must stop inflicting adult interactions on children and making demands that children participate in ways they cannot successfully negotiate. Instead, I encourage clinicians to enter, and direct parents to enter, the world of children, thereby offering them opportunities for rich and reciprocal emotional contact with the adult world.

Merging Spheres

Adults can be viewed as operating in one sphere while children operate in another. Some parents manage to overlap the spheres from time to time as their children mature, whereas other parents experience great distress until their children are mature enough to negotiate interactions in the adult sphere.

How often do parents and other adults become elated when they perceive a child to be capable of holding a conversation with them, or when he/she is finally considered to be a "human being" (meaning the child is older and can communicate verbally and interact on a more mature level)? It appears that younger children's sphere of operation leaves many adults feeling perturbed and alienated, and yet it is productive to bring the spheres into closer proximity so that a compatible coexistance can be developed. The spheres do not necessarily need to repel one another, and yet the most frequent attempt at merger—getting the child to enter the adult's world—is often unsuccessful and unrewarding. A greater success in merging spheres is possible when adults make an effort to infiltrate children's worlds. After all, adults have all been young at one time, hence they have all had experience functioning within the child's sphere. Adults can retrieve some of their earlier thoughts, feelings, sensations, and wonderments, although some adults have an easier time than others reminiscing about their own childhoods, or reexperiencing earlier sensations.

Adults also have cognitive abilities and skills that facilitate tasks such as empathizing with others' feelings and actions. With work, adults can let go of rigid interactional patterns and cognitive styles. Indeed, they have a greater chance of accomplishing this task than children, who have developmental limitations that can restrict their easy entry into adult worlds. Further, the rewards of allowing and encouraging adults to enter children's worlds are without limit. Clinicians will find that the work of therapy is greatly enhanced by encouraging a merging of spheres. By doing so, they are better able to diagnose and then treat behavioral or emotional problems in children.

Play therapists have merged spheres in constant and creative ways. And yet they have often been unable to teach parents the necessary skills, or have focused on teaching parents other important lessons which require them to function as educators, with the result that they maintain a firm footing in the adult world. One of the most optimistic play therapy techniques, called "filial therapy," seeks to engage parents as therapeutic agents, teaching them specific skills to engage and respond to their children in healthy and effective ways. In this type of therapy, developed by Guerney (1964), parents are taught to be empathic, fully accepting of the child, allow the child to play freely, and to convey understanding and acceptance to the child. As a result, parents are empowered to regard themselves as competent in working with their children, as opposed to viewing professionals as the only ones able to manage their children's behavior. Along the same lines, I believe that therapists can teach parents to observe, decode, and *participate* in their children's play in such a way that their understanding of their child's experience is enhanced, and the possibility for deeper emotional contact with their children becomes available. So in addition to the goals of filial therapy described previously, I engage and direct parents to use play techniques, rather than encouraging empathic observation alone.

WHY FOCUS ON CHILDREN'S PLAY?

The reason to focus on children's play is simple and straightforward. Play is the child's medium of communication, hence is replete with opportunities for gaining a deeper understanding of a child and his/her family. Through play, underlying thoughts and feelings are exposed, and children and their families can have collective pleasure and joy at the same time. Play is a universal activity for children, and, as we have seen in

Chapter 1, it has many curative elements. In addition to helping professionals assess children's personality development, self-image, and how they view their worries, concerns, and relational issues, play also grants children the opportunity to solve problems, release tension, discover alternative adaptive behaviors, heal their emotional injuries, and amplify their understanding of the world.

Children will achieve feelings of mastery and control through play. There is general consensus regarding the necessity that children obtain feelings of mastery and competence if they are to achieve a good self-image and positive self-regard. Further, children who suffer painful and potentially traumatic experiences such as abuse, surgery, lengthy hospitalizations, family or community violence, abandonment, parental death, and other difficulties, may use play to help assimilate these stressful experiences and to compensate in fantasy for real losses and difficulties.

THE USE OF PLAY THERAPY TO DIAGNOSE

Clinicians must gather data, obtain a behavioral description of the problem presented and how it affects family members, develop a hypothesis about what is causing and maintaining the problem, and design clinical interventions to ameliorate the problem. When parents come into therapy to discuss their young children's problematic behaviors, it is striking that clinicians will often undertake therapy with the family without seeing or interacting with the young children. Often, parents are asked to bring in their young children only for the perfunctory observation of the child's appearance and superficial interaction with the parents. Further, clinicians have confided their discomfort at these "difficult" sessions, in which the children distract and interrupt the adult dialogue. Assigning a joint task (such as drawing a picture or playing a board game) affords clinicians a first-hand view of how parents organize themselves to enter a joint task, what verbal and nonverbal communication skills they use, and how parents and children negotiate fairness, boredom, limit-setting, and so on. The clinician can also detect issues of relatedness and attachment and other interactional dimensions.

THE USE OF PLAY THERAPY IN FAMILY THERAPY WORK

In addition to providing renewed and ample opportunities for the collection of additional levels of information, play therapy is a useful and dynamic approach in the ongoing treatment of families with young children. Play has the potential to engage all family members in meaningful therapeutic exchanges. When clinicians exclude children, part of the family system remains unengaged, in spite of the fact that some benefit is derived from working with one portion of the family system.

When play is included in family sessions, clinicians treat children as equally important family members, with valuable information to provide and to assimilate. Play is recognized by many therapists as being inherently valuable, because it lowers defenses and elicits and unlocks a deeper level of interaction, in which fantasy, metaphor, and symbol can emerge.

Clinicians also recognize that play can bring people together in a common, pleasurable task, which inherently promotes disinhibition and enjoyment. One parent, who had just participated in a family puppet story (see Chapter 4), was surprised by her own pleasure:

> "At first I thought this was really stupid and I made an effort just for the kids. Slowly, especially when we began the actual acting in the story, I really got into the part of being a lost lamb and a brave soldier. It was fun . . . that's the best way to say it . . . I wasn't just watching the kids play, I was on the floor with a little smile on my face, lost in the play."

When I encouraged this parent to play with her children, not only did I (as the family therapist) learn a lot about their issues based on the story they told, their ability to use play facilitated family relatedness. This experience gave them an opportunity to see each other differently, get into each other's shoes, and laugh together. This positive interaction ended up reaping therapeutic benefits for the following 2 or 3 weeks. Further, because they had all had a positive experience, they subsequently made spontaneous efforts to repeat the family play.

As I will describe in the following sections, play techniques can engage parents and children in enhanced communication, understanding, and emotional relatedness, and can assist clinicians in their important work, and thus should be considered a viable and pivotal part of the family therapy work.

P·A·R·T T·W·O

The Application of Play Therapy Techniques and Clinical Examples

Metaphors can have many different forms. They can be allegories, analogies, similes, proverbs, anecdotes, stories, parables, art, objects (for example, puppets, toy animals, toy trucks), cartoons, poetry, music, and games. . . .

The significant difference between the use of metaphors in therapy and the use of metaphors in other settings is in the goal(s). Metaphors outside of the therapeutic setting, such as stories told by grandparents, or fairy tales, aim to teach specific messages and make definite points. The goal(s) of therapeutic metaphors is to offer new choices, show different ways of perceiving a situation, and tap a variety of dormant beliefs, attitudes and values of the child. The therapist creates individualized metaphors for the child, based on psychodynamic qualities.

—DIANE E. FREY (1993)

F·O·U·R

Family Puppet Interviews

The use of puppets was first promoted by Woltmann (1940) as a valuable technique in helping hospitalized children cope with their illnesses or medical procedures and separation from parents. Others, including Linn (1977) and Alger, Linn, and Beardslee (1985), have also promoted the use of puppets with children in hospital settings. Woltmann found puppets helpful because they are easy to manipulate, offer richness in symbolism, and provide opportunities for spontaneity. Haworth (quoted in Bow, 1993) writes that puppet play "creates an unrealistic and nonthreatening atmosphere that assists in the identification process, thereby encouraging the projection of emotional aspects and interpersonal relationships through the characters" (p. 28). Webb (1991) states that puppets are used in therapy because children identify with the puppets or dolls; project their own feelings onto the play figures; and displace their conflicts onto them, thereby allowing clinicians and children to "talk about feelings or thoughts that 'belong' to the doll or puppet and that the child therefore, does not have to acknowledge as his own" (p. 33). Bow (1993) describes a creative technique called "hidden puppet" to overcome a child's resistance to treatment (p. 27).

Irwin and Shapiro (1975) devised a semistructured puppet interview for assessment purposes; this interview format includes a rating form to assess the content and dimension of story data with a variety of populations (Irwin & Kovacs, 1979; Irwin, Portner, Elmer, & Petti, 1981; Portner, 1981). Irwin (1993) describes the puppet assessment interview as consisting of a "warm-up," in which clinicians bring out puppets and observe children's reactions, inviting their selection of "characters" for their stories; a puppet show, which children develop without the clinician's participation; an interview with the puppets, in which clinicians ask "what" and "why" questions within the realm of the story; and a post-interview with the child, in which the child is invited to discuss the story. Clinicians rate content dimensions such as title, setting, characters, plot, and themes; and form dimensions such as level of creativity, coherence and intelligibility, impulsivity, nonverbal communications, and ego control. In doing so, Irwin maintains that diagnostic data can be derived regarding children's defenses and coping styles, and their preoccupations and conflicts.

The "Family Puppet Interview" (FPI) is described by Irwin and Malloy (1975) as a strategy that stimulates communication and demonstrates how a family mobilizes toward a goal or task. Irwin and Malloy speculate that the use of the FPI puts families at ease, and is particularly effective when there are communication difficulties, or with highly intellectualized or analytical families. Further, the FPI can be used during the diagnostic phase to assess family functioning or during treatment when a specific issue or difficulty arises.

FPIs also create an opportunity for the use of symbolic communication, which can, in turn, become an avenue for conflict resolution and discussion. Symbols provide a safe way for speaking in code. For instance, a child who has used a specific puppet to symbolize her anger (e.g., a shark), may simply reach for the shark when that feeling state occurs.

In addition, FPIs give families a unique way to make contact. During the interviews, family members have fun, alter their tone of voice and physical postures, respond in a unique and spontaneous manner with each other, for instance, with gestures and mannerisms they might never have expressed before within the family. As the stories develop, individuals interact on two levels: content and process. Further, they listen to each other's stories in an effort to create a cohesive story. This obvious cooperation in the creation of a unified story may be a departure from established interactional patterns. A family's inability to organize around a task, interact sufficiently to create and later share a story, may reflect severe dysfunction or conflict, which can alert the clinician to underlying issues.

The FPI is introduced to the family in a matter-of-fact and relaxed way in order to convey that puppet play is a standard therapy technique. Therapists who concern themselves with the family's resistance to this type of work should keep in mind that it is often the clinician's own resistance that creates a systemic hesitancy to proceed with the family intervention. One way I have found to reduce resistance is to tell families at intake that I use a variety of different techniques in working with families, thus it is possible I might ask them to participate in a variety of ways, including art work, puppet play, and story-telling. In this way, families become comfortable with the idea that treatment includes verbal therapy as well as expressive therapies, and thus may feel less self-conscious when they are asked to participate in a broader array of therapies. In addition, families are less likely to feel singled out as requiring a special technique if they understand from the beginning that clinicians will avail themselves of a variety of techniques.

A clinician might introduce puppet play in the following way:

> "I brought some puppets today and I'm going to ask you to take a few minutes and choose the puppets that you would like to work with. Then I'm going to ask you to make up a story with a beginning, a middle, and an end. There are only a couple of rules: You must make up a story, not tell one like Cinderella or Pinocchio, and you must act out the story with your puppets rather than narrate

it. I will give you about 30 minutes to make up the story, and when you are ready you will tell me the story."

These initial interviews usually last a little longer than the typical 50-minute session. An hour and one-half interview is usually an adequate amount of time.

In describing the range of puppets clinicians should make available to child clients, Irwin (1993) says the following:

> In order to gain information about the child's ideas and feelings, a range of puppets must be provided for the child's selection. Fifteen to twenty puppets seem to be enough to provide an adequate selection, with a choice within categories. It is equally important for the puppets to represent a range of affects, including aggressive, friendly, and "neutral" puppets. The selection includes real and fantasy puppets, i.e., realistic family puppets, both black and white (man, woman, boy, girl); royalty family puppets (queen, king, princess, prince); occupational puppets (nurse, doctor, policeman, teacher); symbolic character types (ghost, witch, devil, skeleton, pirate, bum); animal puppets, both wild and tame (dog, bird, monkey, alligator/dragon). Animals should be included, inasmuch as they offer distance and a safe disguise, and are often ready objects for identification. (p. 71)

I believe this selection of puppets is equally useful when working with families. However, clinicians may want to increase the number of puppets to approximately thirty. In addition, I have found it interesting to provide duplicates of selected puppets. In families with blurred boundaries and lack of differentiation, or with cases of sibling rivalry, children or other family members may struggle to be "the same" as others. Hence, with duplicates these issues might be revealed to the therapist.

In addition to the puppets suggested by Irwin (1993), several puppets have been very beneficial in my work with families, in general, and with abused children in particular. They include turtles, with a hard shell to which they can be made to retreat;

tarantulas or other spiders, who have the potential to scare others, and yet can alternately be "good," that is, harmless spiders; sharks, who have the ability to intimidate others and make quick entrances and exits; caterpillars that can turn into butterflies; fairy godmothers, who can grant wishes; judges, who can make decisions; police, who can maintain the laws; and reversible puppets, which can be turned over to uncover another character. In addition, it is useful to have puppets of divergent ethnic backgrounds and skin color, as well as puppets that might provide specific cultural symbolism (such as indigenous healers, priests, mariachis, and so on).

Once family members select their puppets, clinicians can observe them through a one-way mirror as they make up their stories. This process is important to watch because it demonstrates and clarifies how the family organizes to undertake and complete a task. Clinicians should assess who starts the story and who introduces what themes; how the puppets are assigned or shared; who is intrusive with their themes or decisions; who follows and who leads; whether there are family collusions or alliances; who is pessimistic about the task and how others respond; who power resides with; how decisions are made; etc. If one-way mirrors are not available, clinicians can either sit in the room unobtrusively to observe the process, or they can leave the room and videotape the family's preparation of the story. Whether the family is being observed in the room by the clinician, videotaped, or viewed by the clinician or others behind a one-way mirror, it is necessary to obtain the permission of the family and answer all questions about the nature of the observation or recording. Because young children cannot give informed consent, their parents hold that privilege and can consent on the children's behalf. However, I believe it is important to explain recording or observation procedures to children in simple language, answer all their questions or concerns beforehand, and allow them to give their permission, although in reality that permission is not necessary once parental consent is obtained.

If the session is videotaped, tapes can serve as educational tools with the family later on. Families have often told me how enjoyable and informative it is to observe their story-telling, and that they have had many insights into their own behavior by watching the taped session. Clinicians observe and document throughout the FPI. In particular, therapists note which puppets are selected by family members since these choices provide important information. Puppets are chosen for idiosyncratic reasons, which are either immediately obvious or later understood. The themes introduced by family members are also important to record, as well as which themes become dominant and which are obscured during the family's story.

When the family has decided upon its story, the clinician asks for each person to introduce his/her puppet with a name if one has been assigned, and then say a couple of sentences about the puppet. Once the introductions of puppets are made, the therapist discourages narration of the story by saying, "Don't tell me about what the puppet says, let the puppets speak for themselves." It is worth noting that children will more naturally enter the roles of their puppets and stay within those roles. Sometimes adults have difficulty with taking the first person, and thus may prefer instead to say things like "then he wasn't sure how he felt and he asked his friend to come over to play." The clinician at this point might intervene and role-model, "I'm not sure how I feel. Mr. Crow, can you come over and play with me?" Indeed, the therapist may need to correct or intervene until the family becomes engaged in the play. Clinicians can also clarify meaning by talking directly to the puppets.

Once the story is complete, Irwin and Malloy (1975) direct the clinician to ask questions about the story, and invite discussion by asking each family member to give a title (or name) to the story, as well as to explain the moral or lesson of the story. Each family member is also asked to tell which puppet they would most and least like to be.

One variation I have found useful, prior to the cognitive task of discussing the story, is for the clinician to enter the family's story by directing interaction between characters, eliciting dialogue, or asking for clarification or expansion of the story. In this way the magic of the family's metaphor is not interrupted by the clinician's focus on distanced observation, retrospection, or interpretation. Therefore, before asking for the family's feedback, which naturally changes the dynamics of the play active during the story-telling, I believe it is useful for the clinician to employ a variety of interactions such as the following:

1. Determine the content or theme of the story, and then reframe it so as to create meanings that might become helpful in the therapy.

2. Create new interactions within the context of the family's metaphor. For instance, with two puppets who have not spoken (reflecting family conflict or distance), the therapist might ask the puppets to consider a question together, or share their experiences or feelings with one another.

3. Wonder out loud. When a conflict or a situation is introduced into the story, wonder out loud about whether there were other instances in which that conflict was present and what the puppets remember about those times.

4. Pose questions. Ask puppets to consider specific questions about their or other puppet's behaviors or feelings. Go beyond what has been reported by the family and allow them to consider new explanations.

5. Challenge. The clinician may find an opportunity to challenge a belief system (or outcome) displayed in the story. The clinician can challenge the story-telling system to further explain or resolve.

6. As with the Mutual Story-Telling Technique (see Chapter 6), the clinician postulates about the outcome of the story: Do the puppets resolve conflict in a positive, healthy manner? Does the outcome need to be reconsidered? The clinician can introduce other, more positive, outcomes and ask the family to consider these options.

7. Comment on the story-telling system. The clinician can reflect a family's ambivalence by noting that half of the family is of one mind, while half of the family is of another mind. He/she should then consider how these conflicts will be resolved?

8. Look for "exceptions": Using Michael White's concept of narrative therapy, I will often ask about "exceptions" to the themes presented in the family's story. For example, if the story includes a withdrawn or absent father, I may direct family members, in character, to provide information on times the parent is present and available and what interactions and reactions occur in these situations. In this way, White proposes, individuals expand on their life stories, integrating information relegated to nonimportant because it has been excluded from thought (White & Epston, 1990).

Once the clinician has "entered" the family's metaphor, and explored, challenged, questioned, and encouraged ongoing interactions, he/she can bring the family out of the metaphor by posing the questions mentioned earlier, regarding title, moral of the story, which puppet family members would most/least like to be, and, finally, whether each family member sees any relationship between the family's problems or difficulties and the story they told.

This technique can be very powerful and can successfully change therapy that has become flat or stifled, in which individuals remain disconnected and uncommunicative, use rigid or superficial communication, or prefer intellectualized reasoning that has not facilitated dynamic change.

CASE ILLUSTRATION 1

Lucy was a single Caucasian mother who had lived alone with her two young daughters for the past 6 years. In the 6 months prior to coming to therapy, she had met a man, fallen in love, and invited him to live with her and her daughters. The two girls, Ashley, age 8, and Caren, 10, had had a very difficult time with this change. They had become sullen, incommunicative, and, most distressing to their mother, prone to violent temper outbursts with each other and their friends. Further, their school work had deteriorated acutely, and they had begun to exhibit aggressive behaviors while in school. They also had refused to do household chores, and seemed to purposely be provocative around their new house guest, Jim. Jim was a divorced man of Irish descent who had raised five children of his own who were now in their 20s. He was authoritarian and felt it was his job to be a father figure to the two girls, whom he described as "unruly." He did not find it easy to communicate and preferred to "carry a big stick." Lucy deferred all authority to him, and apparently despaired at her daughters' embarrassing behaviors. She had been raised by a strict father and thus found Jim's behavior quite familiar. She saw his attempts to discipline the children as a symbol of his love for her and commitment to the relationship at great personal sacrifice.

The First Session: The Initial Interview

I asked Lucy to bring Jim and her children to the first session, in which I could gather information from everyone about the problem. Jim was unwilling to attend because he did not believe in therapy; his previous marital relationship had ended in spite of 1 year of therapy, and, as he described it, "because" of therapy. "Some things are better left alone," he quipped to his live-in partner. Lucy was tearful as she described how the girls had changed, how selfish they had become, and how she felt scared that Jim might leave her if she could not get the girls to behave.

Both girls were flat and unresponsive. Their crossed arms and lowered heads did not belie their feelings; they were angry and hurt. They could not control what their mom was doing, but they could control whether they spoke to me or not. That first session consisted of my talking to Lucy, my encouraging her to tell me about the two girls, particularly how they behaved prior to Jim's moving in, and my obtaining more information about their background. I learned that Lucy's husband, Patrick, had abandoned her with little fanfare. She had come home one night to find all of his clothes and personal belongings gone. There had been no note, no goodbye, no nothing. She described being in a state of shock for months since she had not anticipated his departure and had not been aware of his unhappiness in the marriage. She described the stress of finding herself left with two very young children and a low-paying job. She had become very depressed but felt that she had to forge ahead for the sake of her young children. Although the situation had been "rough," she felt that it had helped the girls and herself become a closer family; she had spent all of her free time with the girls watching favorite sports events or taking them out to movies or shopping. Lucy noted that both girls had been cooperative, and had volunteered to help around the house prior to Jim's moving in. Also, everyone had seemed to be getting along— there had been typical sibling squabbling and fighting over clothes and other things, but nothing as unpleasant and violent as it had become lately.

Lucy said that Jim was a very nice, decent, hard-working man. She added, "They should thank their lucky stars that he's patient with them—any other man would have packed his bags and run as fast as he could." (This seemed like a covert reference to the girls' father.) As I have already noted, the girls were unresponsive to their mother's tears, accusations, and general despair, as if they had made an agreement to pursue a steady course of disagreeable behavior. By the end of the session, I empathized with the mother's frustration: The girls were definitely a powerful team, standing firmly united and silent.

The Second Session: The Family Puppet Interview

In the second session, the two girls dragged in with defiant looks and clear passive aggressive body language. Jim was once again absent. I escorted the three of them into a therapy room in which I had placed about 12 puppets on a table in the room's center. The girls looked at them with restrained curiosity.

"Today we'll be doing something different," I began. "I would like each of you to look at the puppets on the table and notice the ones that are the most interesting to you. I'd like you to then choose the ones you would like to use to tell me a story that has a beginning, middle, and end." The girls moved away from the table and sank into their chairs, thereby expressing noncompliance. I continued:

"There are only a few rules. First of all, you have to make up a story together, the three of you, that has a beginning, middle, and end, and it has to be a made-up story, not something like Cinderella or Pinocchio. Secondly, once you are ready to tell your story you act it out with your puppets, you don't just narrate the story. I will leave the room and let you discuss the story you want to tell, and I'll rejoin you in about 30 minutes or sooner, if you just go over and open the door to signal that you are ready to tell the story."

In the first session I had informed them that I audiotape sessions and asked for their signed permission to do so. The audiotape was on, therefore, to record their preparation of the story. As I left the room there was a long silence. Finally, the older girl said, "This is stupid. I don't want to do this. I hate coming here. I wanna go." Her younger sister, as expected from Lucy's description of acute sibling rivalry, took the opposite point of view: "You're stupid that's what! And you don't know any good stories anyway." The mother, showing a flash of brilliance, refused to take sides and simply stated, "I don't like the idea of playing with puppets, but maybe there's something to this that we'll enjoy." As I left the room, it was clear that the family had bonded in an effort to make the task as painless as possible. After a long pause, some choices were made. Mother grabbed the police officer puppet. The younger girl chose a rabbit and a squirrel, while the older girl chose a bear and an owl. They began to construct the story, although mother had to intervene often since the girls became argumentative about the direction of the story. The girls argued less about content and more about control, that is, who would remain in charge of where the story went. You could hear the mother's frustration mount when the girls quibbled with each other. Finally, she withdrew and restrained from attempting to stop the bickering. As she did, the girls became more cooperative and appeared to be enjoying the process of creating a story. The mother's contribution to the story was minimal—she had removed herself from the process in frustration and the girls had not invited her to participate. Putting the story together reflected the process of division taking place at home, in which the girls teamed up against their mother (and Jim).

After 15 minutes, the girls signaled that they had completed their task by opening the door. I entered the room and sat across from the family. The girls seemed as energized as the mother seemed deflated. I asked them to tell me their story. Caren began by saying, "I am a wise old owl, the oldest in this jungle, and I'm here to report that there's some trouble brewing below." She burst into laughter upon hearing the deep voice she had chosen to represent the owl. "I hear lots of noise coming from that house over there, and someone else can tell you more." She looked at her mother, and motioned it was her turn to speak. Mother said, "I am the police officer and I patrol this street, and I'm here to tell you there's some pretty wild stuff going on in some of these houses. Why, in that house yonder, just last night, someone called me to come over and stop a disturbance of the peace."

There was a pause and Caren motioned to Ashley to begin. "I don't like living here," said Ashley. "I live in a tree outside the top bedroom window. And I can look in and see all the mean and loud people. Sometimes I just run away to see my friends in other trees where it is more quiet." Ashley then brought out her other hand with the rabbit puppet. "And I like to jump around; I jump high, high, high, higher than most rabbits my size. And when I jump sometimes I get up so high

I can look inside windows and sometimes kids are watching TV and sometimes they are getting spanked. I jump, jump, jump into the next yard when the kids get spanked a lot and a lot." Mother piped in with: "My job is to keep the peace in the neighborhood and to make sure that the squirrels and rabbits can feel safe and comfortable in the front yards. My job is to make sure people are getting along and that the rules are not being broken." Caren added: "Sometimes the policeman doesn't get there in time and then we have some bloody fights. When the police comes and asks questions, they get lies and more lies and then they don't know something bad is going on. Sometimes the police are plain stupid and don't get it at all."

Ashley's squirrel spoke up: "It's not the policeman's fault all the time. Sometimes the people lie to the police and tell them everything is alright when it's not." Caren concluded with, "I am the bear and I can tell you that is why I have to hibernate. I need a break from all the crazy people. I just go and sleep and sleep. When I wake up sometimes things are better. Other times I might have to come and step on top of the houses and tear them down. That's how mad I can get with people who keep bothering me." Ashley then says: "The end."

After relating the story, Caren and Ashley put their puppets back on the table and sat back in their chairs. Lucy held on to the police officer puppet. The following dialogue then ensued:

THERAPIST: It seems to me there is a lot of fighting going on in this story and everybody doesn't like it. I wonder what all the fighting is about?

POLICE OFFICER (mother): It seems to me that people have forgotten how to get along.

THERAPIST: Specifically, Mrs. Police Officer, who doesn't get along?

POLICE OFFICER (mother): Inside the houses, the people who live there, they have forgotten to get along.

THERAPIST: Mr. Owl, oh wisest and eldest of owls, why do you think people have forgotten to get along?

OWL (Caren): (*Slipping the owl back on her hand*) Because sometimes everything is fine and then somebody mean comes along and ruins everything, and then everything is yucky.

THERAPIST: What do you think, Mr. Squirrel, you who can climb tall trees and look inside?

SQUIRREL (Ashley): I think the owl said it.

THERAPIST: You agree with the owl?

SQUIRREL (Ashley): Mean people ruin things.

THERAPIST: Mr. Owl, what mean people do you know?

OWL (Caren): Mostly big, fat, hairy men!

RABBIT (Ashley): They try to chase us but we run faster, ha, ha.

THERAPIST: So both the rabbit and the owl know mean people who are men.

BEAR (Caren): I will trample over them with my big and smelly feet.

THERAPIST: Mrs. Police Officer, what do you think about big, fat, and hairy men who chase after rabbits?

POLICE OFFICER (mother): I think that sometimes even though they are big and fat and hairy, they are not mean, and sometimes if people didn't run away, they would get to see that.

OWL (Caren): Oh, sure, oh sure, you know better. The big, hairy, fat men are nice; we creatures of the animal kingdom don't know what we're talking about (*in defiant tone*).

POLICE OFFICER (mother): I think you know a lot. But sometimes people are not mean, they just make a lot of noise, like the lion who growls in the jungle. He's not always mean; he just has a habit of growling.

OWL (Caren): Oh, yes. The lions growl to be friendly . . . they want to be your best friend so they can eat you up for dessert after you trust them.

POLICE OFFICER (mother): But sometimes the lions are friendly and they won't eat you up or hurt you.

RABBIT (Ashley): If a lion ate me, I would kick his stomach with my big paws and I would give him a stomach ache.

THERAPIST: You would keep fighting no matter what happened.

RABBIT (Ashley): Because my feet are big and strong.

THERAPIST: And, Mr. Bear, you would stomp over anybody who tried to hurt you?

BEAR (Caren): Stomp them because I'm bigger.

THERAPIST: It sounds like everyone is busy protecting themselves. What do you think you can do to help, Mrs. Police Officer?

POLICE OFFICER (mother): Sometimes I think I can't do much. There's only one of me. Everybody calls for help at the same time. Nobody seems to trust anyone anymore.

THERAPIST: And how does that make you feel?

POLICE OFFICER (mother): I just get wiped out. Exhausted. Sometimes I just want to give up. (*Tears start rolling down her cheeks.*)

THERAPIST: Mr. Owl, you are wise and all-knowing, as well as sensitive to other's feelings, what can you say to Mrs. Police Officer?

OWL (Caren): Well . . . I don't know. It's a tough job. You have to listen to everybody and not be fooled by people who tell you everything is alright because it's not. What do you think, Mr. Squirrel?

SQUIRREL (Ashley): (*Ashley moves physically closer and has the squirrel puppet cuddle up to the police officer puppet.*) There, there, don't be sad. I can help you. You can come to my treehouse sometime and share some of my nuts. I have plenty.

Caren interrupts the story by asking if it is time to go yet. I respond that we have about 5 minutes.

THERAPIST: Mrs. Police Officer, what do you think is the title of your story?

POLICE OFFICER (mother): "Watching the Beat Makes Me Tired."

THERAPIST: What's your title, Mr. Owl?

OWL (Caren): "The Owl Knows."

THERAPIST: What's your title, Mr. Bear?

BEAR (Caren): "Sleep It Off."

THERAPIST: What's your title, Mr. Squirrel?

SQUIRREL (Ashley): "Nuts Are Plenty."

THERAPIST: And what's your title, Mr. Rabbit?

RABBIT (Ashley): "Big Feet Are Best."

THERAPIST: Thank you everyone for telling me your story. I learned a lot from listening, especially how you all seem to be in the same boat: You know there's a lot of fighting going on, you don't know how to make it stop, and you all understand how hard it is for the police officer to listen to everyone and try to help.

This week, before I see you again, I'd like you to do the following homework: Mr. Police Officer, take the owl out for a quiet walk with just the two of you, and simply listen to whatever the owl has to tell you. Mr. Owl, you have so much to say; don't say it all at once, but tell the police officer some of what you've been learning by watching over everyone.

Mr. Police Officer, I'd like you also to take Mr. Squirrel up on her invitation to share her nuts. Let her escort you to wherever she would like to go to share some of her favorite nuts. You don't have to talk about anything in particular, just share your nuts together.

And now I have a special homework task for Mr. Bear and Mr. Rabbit. Instead of stomping and kicking, I'd like you to use your strength and quickness in some other ways, and I'd like you to watch the big, hairy, fat man from afar, and just notice if he does anything at all that's not mean. You might have to watch long and hard to *catch him* doing something that's not mean, but your job is to watch and listen, listen and watch .

And now it's time to stop. I'll see you all next week at the same time.

Commentary

The children's resistance to creating a family puppet story was brief. I stated my expectations of the task simply and without discussion. Sometimes I have supervised clinicians who use this technique and seem to ask for the parent's permission in such an ambivalent way that families sense the clinician's discomfort and choose not to comply. For example, they may say, "Would you be willing to do this?" or "There's something I'd like you to consider." When children are involved, it's always best to present a task as a fait accompli, rather than offering them opportunities to decline.

Also, I presented the directions succinctly and without too much complication. Sometimes I hear directives that are too long and complex for children to understand. If there are too many rules, the game may not sound conducive to play. Hence, there are only two rules: The story must be made up, and it must be acted out (not narrated).

Leaving the room as soon as possible, after giving instructions, forces the family to unite to complete a task. If there is resistance, the clinician usually becomes the target of the resistance. Sometimes the family division can be observed as the task is undertaken, as with this family, who exhibited the very issue they encountered at home: The children became combative and the mother retreated in frustration thereby perpetuating the children's ongoing collusion against the parents. At home, the mother's withdrawal represented a signal to her boyfriend to assist her, hence he entered the scenario to get the girls' combative behavior under control and thereby protect the mother. With the boyfriend's absence in the therapy session, the mother's retreat eventually elicited the girls' cooperation with each other but perpetuated the separation between the parent and her children.

The children made interesting choices in puppets. It is significant that the older daughter Caren chose to be the wise owl and the strong and potentially destructive bear. She most likely chose the owl because she was the oldest child and because her opinions had lately been overlooked. She most likely chose the bear as a representative of her strength and immovable position, as well as her ability to be alternately hurtful and nurturing to those around her. Ashley chose the quick and strong rabbit as well as the squirrel, who has observing and nesting instincts. Both a squirrel and a rabbit are quick to scurry when trouble appears. Resembling these animals, Ashley herself was known for running around the house to escape from her older sister's loud threats, and for finding refuge in small hiding places. The mother also made her obvious best choice, the police officer, since that was the role she described herself as assuming in the household in the first session. In other words, she saw herself as someone who was trying to keep the peace. Indeed, it was interesting to see her police officer puppet despair as more and more people called for help and she found herself unable to be of assistance.

The theme in the story reflected the family's distress: The mother was trying to keep peace between Jim, who was perceived as a potential threat, and the children, who either ran from him or attacked him verbally. Both children displayed observational skills and their accumulated knowledge that men are unreliable and frightening. They also both exemplified their willingness to fight to the finish rather than accept what they believed to be a dangerous fate.

In the process of fighting, many things had been lost. The children were so intent on self-protection that they had built a protective wall around them: Nothing hurt them, but the wall also kept out any potential positive interactions. In building the protective wall, they not only kept out the potential threat, Jim, they also kept out the police officer, their mother. The fact that they bonded together to fight off the perceived threat also strengthened their sense of being unprotected by mother.

My interventions were designed to encourage some emotional exchange between each child and her mother. At the same time, I directed the girls to use their observational skills to take in new information about Jim: My statement "See if you can catch him doing something positive" was a challenge to their observational skills. Giving them the task of observing was also intended to divert them from the attack mode. When they left, I felt the family puppet session had been far more effective than the previous session, and I pondered how to get Jim to attend future sessions since he was an integral part of the family dynamic and problem formation.

The Third Session

The following week the girls greeted me more openly and skirted in front of me to the therapy room, apparently anxious to get started. Their mother seemed unchanged and followed behind as we entered the room. The girls asked for the puppets immediately, and I told them I would be happy to bring them out but first I wanted to hear how their week had been. Caren and Ashley said, "Fine" and "Okay" almost simultaneously. Mother added, "Things started off really well after we left here. . . ." I asked her in what way things were good when they had left. Mother reported that the girls seemed more cooperative with each other, and that there were fewer fights for the first 4 or 5 days. "Wow," I replied, "4 or 5 days . . . that's tremendous!" "Yeah, but then all hell broke loose," she continued, "because Ashley asked Jim to help her with her homework and Caren was in a tizzy."

THERAPIST: So, Ashley, you gave Jim a chance to help you out.

ASHLEY: Well, he knows about math stuff.

THERAPIST: So you had observed that he knew about math.

ASHLEY: Yeah, and Caren told me to get out of her room when I asked her for help.

CAREN: I didn't know you'd go ask him.

ASHLEY: Well, he helped me more than you.

CAREN: Shithead!

MOTHER: Caren, watch your language.

CAREN: Well, she is.

MOTHER: See what I mean.

THERAPIST: Sounds like Caren doesn't much like Jim stepping in on her territory.

CAREN: Damn straight.

MOTHER: Caren, one more four-letter word out of you and—

CAREN: And what? You'll get monster Jim to come yell at me?

THERAPIST: What would you do if Jim talked to you instead of your mom?

CAREN: I hate that! I hate that more than anything! She's the one who's our mom. She's the one who's supposed to tell us what's what. Not him. He's nobody. He's not my dad. He can't tell me what to do.

THERAPIST: You don't like it when your mom doesn't speak for herself.

CAREN: I hate it! She's like a wimpy mouse.

THERAPIST: And if she's like a mouse, how's Jim?

CAREN: He's like a huge, stomping . . . tiger, who eats his young and roars and roars—

MOTHER: Caren, you are exaggerating so much. He does not roar and roar.

CAREN: Oh yeah, but he does eat his young right?

MOTHER: No, I didn't say that.

THERAPIST: Caren, are you worried that Jim could gobble all of you up?

CAREN: Yeah.

MOTHER: I don't know what that means.

THERAPIST: Caren, tell your mom what you're worried about.

CAREN: (*Wiping away a tear*) That he's gonna take over. . . . (*She is crying visibly now and stumbling over her words.*) That he'll be in charge of us, and you, and we'll never be the way we were before.

THERAPIST: How have things changed?

CAREN: Before you liked us better—

MOTHER: (*Impatiently*) Caren, don't be ridiculous—

THERAPIST: Lucy, try to listen to how your daughter feels right now, not whether or not the feeling is correct.

CAREN: You used to spend time with us, play games with us, go out with us, now everything is Jim. . . . You treat him like he was your favorite.

THERAPIST: (*Turning to mother*) What feelings do you hear Caren describing to you?

MOTHER: It sounds like she thinks that I spend too much time—

THERAPIST: Lucy, stay with the feelings, how do you think Caren feels?

MOTHER: Lonely, like I don't care . . . unloved, I guess.

THERAPIST: Caren, does that sound about right?

CAREN: Yeah—

THERAPIST: Ashley, you've been listening carefully, is there any other feeling you think Caren has?

ASHLEY: She's scared.

THERAPIST: Scared of what?

ASHLEY: Losing mommy.

THERAPIST: And you, Ashley? How do you feel?

ASHLEY: I feel scared too.

THERAPIST: What are you scared about?

ASHLEY: That mommy will go away and be with Jim all the time.

THERAPIST: Anything else?

ASHLEY: That she'll go away like daddy did.

THERAPIST: You're worried she'll go away and not return?

ASHLEY: Yeah.

THERAPIST: Mom, what do you hear your children saying?

MOTHER: That they're worried I'll leave like their dad. . . . (*Mom is crying now too.*) But I need them to know—

THERAPIST: Tell them directly.

MOTHER: I will never, never leave you—well, not unless I die, or when I die, but that won't be of my own free will.

THERAPIST: Tell them how you feel about them.

MOTHER: Don't you know how much I love you girls?

THERAPIST: Tell them.

MOTHER: I love you more than anything or anybody.

CAREN: More than Jim?

MOTHER: Of course more than Jim. You were here before him and you will be in my life forever, and no matter what happens with Jim, you will always be my girls.

THERAPIST: When was the last time all of you hugged each other?

MOTHER: They don't seem to like being kissed and hugged anymore.

THERAPIST: When was the last time?

MOTHER: Months ago.

THERAPIST: About 7 months or so?

MOTHER: Yeah, about that.

THERAPIST: My impression is that most children like to be hugged and kissed even when they get bigger and older.

MOTHER: Would you kids like a hug?

Ashley responded to her mother's open arms immediately. Caren watched as they hugged. Mother opened her arms further to include Caren and Caren moved into the hug as Ashley moved to her mother's side. I told them to enjoy their hug as long as they wanted. The mother sat holding her children for about 15 minutes and as they started to move about I asked them where they were going to go right after the session. Caren said that Ashley and her mom had found a new ice cream store, and that mom had promised them a treat before they had dinner.

I told them I hoped they would have a nice treat before dinner, and that the only homework for the following week would be to try hugging two more times, but not more than two times,* and to continue to keep watching Jim to see if they still could catch him doing something that was not mean. Ashley could not resist telling me that she had caught him twice already. I told her to write the two things down so she would not forget them and that we could talk about him next week. On her way out, Ashley said, "We forgot to play with the puppets." "Yeap we did," I replied, "they'll be here next time."

---

* I obviously did not want to limit family hugging but recognized this was currently unfamiliar behavior and perhaps not easy to reproduce outside the therapy. Therefore, I gave a paradoxical intervention in the hope it would relieve anxiety and elicit the family's rebelliousness (i.e., "We'll hug as often as we want"). For additional description of paradoxical interventions, see Palazzoli, Boscolo, Cecchin, & Prata, 1981.

Commentary

This had been a successful session. I was surprised at how much had been accomplished so quickly, but I credited the mother for bringing the children to therapy at just the right moment. They were showing signs of distress, but they had not yet gotten into rigid patterns of behavior. Underneath the surface, the children were desperately seeking the attention of their mother. The fact that their father had deserted them very early in life, and that their mother had developed a compliant response vis-à-vis her relationship with Jim, threatened the children's sense of security and heightened their fears of abandonment.

My primary goal was to reestablish the emotional bond that had existed prior to Jim's arrival. Luckily, there was much to draw from, unlike with some families where the conflict has caused deep divisive rifts between family members. I relied on the fact that if the emotional bond could be reestablished, other problems could be tackled more easily.

This family was undergoing a severe emotional crisis because of Jim's presence. The girls had to adjust to him as someone their mother loved, had to renegotiate the amount of time they spent with their mother, and had to accept his authority as a father figure. Mother and Jim had some unresolved issues as well. In an effort to hold onto the relationship, Lucy had lost her voice. She delegated authority over the children to Jim, without attempting to establish equal parenting. Her behavior was motivated by the fear of being abandoned by a man she could not make happy. She had not anticipated the breakup of her former marriage, and therefore went to great lengths to ensure that Jim was content and satisfied, often sacrificing her own preferences and choices.

Jim had noticed that there was an improvement around the house and had told Lucy he was happy she had had better luck in therapy than he had. He still refused to come into therapy, but he acquiesced to Caren's request that he attend one of the sessions. Caren had arrived at the conclusion on her own that Jim was needed in the therapy and decided that she would invite him herself. Jim was so taken aback by Caren's invitation that he decided to attend one single session in which the girls were able to tell him that they had caught him being nice in many, many ways. Ashley brought her book, which listed 14 different items.

Caren set the tone for the session by thanking him for coming to the session even though he did not believe in therapy. She went on to ask him simply to listen to some of the things they wanted to tell him and used her owl to explain how her mother's tendency to take care of Jim exclusively made her feel. Ashley had established a more warm relationship with Jim (as reported by her mother). As a result, she took her squirrel puppet and constantly motioned for Jim's attention, which he provided without being distracted from what Caren had to say. He seemed like a responsive parent figure, eager to fit in with this family. After listening, he said he understood how hard his moving in had been and thanked them for giving him a chance. He added, "Haven't you noticed how I don't go around yelling all the time anymore?" "That's because you two aren't running around like little hoodlums anymore." He then thanked them for their trust and for inviting him to the session. They discussed additional minor problems that had surfaced, but mostly this session felt like one in which the family was formally acknowledging Jim's place in the family. At one point when Jim was expressing his understanding of the children and their discomfort and distrust, he said, "Sometimes my bark is louder than my bite." The girls responded, "Your roar is louder than your gobble."

Conclusion

The FPI was a valuable strategy with the highly incommunicative and hostile children described above. The presenting problem was the children's aggressive behavior which had surfaced when mother's boyfriend had moved into the home. Mother and children had enjoyed a close and warm relationship, which had quickly deteriorated as mother became compliant in an effort to appease her boyfriend. The children perceived mother's boyfriend as a threat and secretly worried that she would leave them for him. Since the children had experienced their own father's abandonment, their fear of their mother's disappearance was understandable.

The children responded well to the FPI and the initial story they presented with underscored their primary problem: The children had developed aggressive postures as a defense against the perceived threat. As they shut out all potential harm from Jim, they also shut out any potential positive interactions. The animals in the story (symbolic of the sibling's primary feelings) frequently either ran, hid, or fought.

The first task was to use the metaphors in the story to encourage contact between mother and children. For instance, the story revealed that Lucy's policing role would need to be replaced by a nurturing role to reinstate positive contact. If the warm contact between mother and children could be reestablished, it was likely that other problems could be tackled. The metaphors from this initial story were brought up throughout the therapy, which lasted for about 6 months. Although Jim attended only one session, the metaphor that appeared of a roar that was louder than a gobble represented the children's fear of being yelled at and being swallowed up. This metaphor became a code that was employed to diffuse arguments. Once metaphors are established with a family, they are available for reference or expansion throughout the therapy. On occasion, I would refer to the squirrel to allude to nesting instincts, or to the bear to allude to our ability to stomp and our ability to be powerful just by being still.

It is unknown how slowly or quickly verbal therapy that did not include play would have proceeded, but it can be said that the play broke through the family's initial resistance and provided rich symbolism with which to work. Many clinicians have expressed hesitancy to engage the families in puppet work apparently because they feel discomfort with the use of play. I believe that in doing so clinicians often stifle their own creative energies, as well as their capacity to have fun and communicate through symbols rather than words. Many of these clinicians have expressed fear over not knowing what to do or say once a family completes its story, and/or the possibility of misinterpreting the story's meaning. Asking questions can help the clinician better understand the story's potential meaning; and once clinicians allow themselves opportunities to practice this technique, they will feel more comfortable to hypothesize regarding the meaning inherent in puppet selection, themes, and interactions within the story.

Clinicians who feel hesitant about using this technique can practice working with family stories with colleagues. This can be done by practically any group of people, although preexisting relationships amongst group members will result in a greater use of symbolism than with newly-formed groups with little common history. Staff members of a group practice can certainly be asked to convene for the purpose of developing and then telling a puppet story. In this way, clinicians can practice what they would say or do as the group story evolves.

Another positive aspect of this technique is that clinicians can provide interventions using their own theoretical frameworks. For example, a clinician well-versed in narrative therapy techniques or Gestalt therapy can use these unique perspectives in family puppet interviews.

CASE ILLUSTRATION 2

Xavier was a 7-year-old South American boy brought to therapy by a frustrated parent, who had placed the child on a diet when he was 4 years old and had felt increasingly helpless as she watched Xavier's steady weight gain. The child was as visibly overweight as his mother was visibly concerned about his appearance. In her first phone call to me she described feeling "at the end of her rope," and remarked that she hoped therapy might help this child lose weight. When I asked about her family, she stated that she was married to a nice, but quiet, husband. Throughout our brief conversation, she referred to her husband,

Tony, as somewhat "disinterested and uninvolved" with the family due to his busy and demanding work. Mother had another child, Monica, who was 6 years old, of normal weight, and a "perfect angel." I invited everyone in the family to attend the first family session and mother reluctantly agreed, though she stated her husband would probably not attend. I told her that it was very important to me that he attend the therapy since as Xavier's father I was sure there was much he could tell me about his son. Mother seemed reluctant but finally agreed to see what she could do to encourage Tony's attendance.

The First Session: The Initial Interview

When I went out to welcome the family in the waiting room, I found that the father was missing. Mother held her daughter Monica in her lap, and Xavier was jumping up and down and making quite a bit of noise. She stood up and shook my hand while saying, "Hi, I'm Fernanda and Tony's outside killing himself slowly . . . I'll get him." Father put out his cigarette and came in the front door as the mother motioned for him. I greeted Tony, telling him how happy I was that he had decided to come since I knew he would be able to tell me a lot about his son. He muttered, "We'll see . . . I don't really know a lot."

In the office, mother again took Monica in her lap, and Monica put her fingers in her mouth, and looked as if she were sitting in her most comfortable and familiar spot. Xavier did not sit but preferred to wander around the room, much to his mother's discomfort. As mother kept telling Xavier to sit down and not touch things, father was quiet, apparently being used to her attempts to structure their son's behavior.

I first ascertained their preferred language for use in the session, and they picked Spanish. We talked for a few minutes about some difficulty they had had in finding the office. I then asked the family to tell me what brought them to therapy. Tony looked at Fernanda and she immediately took the lead: "As I told you on the phone, we are very worried about Xavier's eating and the fact that he keeps gaining weight." As she made this opening statement, Xavier made loud blowing noises with his mouth, and Monica giggled while a fleeting smile crossed Tony's face. Mother continued without responding to Xavier. "He doesn't seem to take it very seriously. . . ." I interrupted by asking if she meant Xavier or Tony. She said, "Xavier of course. He thinks this is some kind of joke but it isn't. He needs to understand that if he doesn't begin to pay attention it's going to get harder and harder to lose weight. I know. I've been overweight all my life and I know how cruel people can be." Xavier interrupted by stating, "Nobody makes fun of me. If they do I'll beat their butts." Mother quickly responded, "Fighting is not going to solve your problem." "I don't have a problem," Xavier yelled. "Who has the problem?", I asked. "I don't know," Xavier yelled back, holding his hands on the back of the couch and kicking his legs up, much as a donkey or horse kicks backward.

Mother was not successful in getting Xavier to sit down. His behavior escalated as I commented on how distracting it was. Mother said that Xavier had always been "hyper" and "disobedient." Father made very few comments and only spoke when spoken to, which did not happen very often. When I turned my attention to him to inquire what he thought about coming to therapy, he referred back to his wife. When I insisted on getting his point of view, he reluctantly and ratherly quietly said, "He gets in a lot of fights because the other boys bother him a lot." When I asked Tony who this was a problem for, he said "mostly Fern" (i.e., his wife). When I asked if Xavier's weight affected him in any way, Tony stated that "things would be more quiet at home if Fern and Xavier weren't always fighting about what he eats." Tony added that he had been a "chubby boy too," due to all "the good food his mom made when he was a child." Mother spoke up: "Good food! All that fat and fried food . . . all those potatoes and rice and desserts! People know better than to cook like that anymore." Father listened quietly. Monica said nothing and sucked her fingers throughout the first 30 minutes of discussion. Xavier opened and closed doors and drawers; ripped leaves from plants; spit; and made loud grunts and yelled, and seemed generally out of control. I decided to cut the session short because of the escalating disruption and the family's frustration and discomfort. I speculated the chaos was reflective of the family's typical difficulties and decided to invite them to return for a different intervention the following week. I told the parents that I had gained a great deal of information from this first meeting and wanted to schedule a second meeting later in the week.

The Second Session: The Family Puppet Interview

The second session took place 2 days later. From the start, Xavier made his presence known in the waiting room. Indeed, two other therapists came out to the waiting room to ask him to keep quiet. Mother acted intolerant and was feeling inadequate and father was chain smoking outside. When the family members entered the room, they saw about 15 puppets on the coffee table in the middle of the room. Xavier seemed earnestly interested in the puppets, asking, "What are these for?" "Well thanks for asking Xavier. These are puppets for you and your family." Xavier looked at me again, and said, "What do you mean?" I sat down and asked them to sit down and get comfortable. "I've brought the puppets today because I want to ask you all to make up a story with these puppets." Monica got out of her mother's lap and sat with her brother around the coffee table.

"What I want each of you to do is to pick out a puppet that you want to work with, a puppet you like, or one that grabs your attention for whatever reason." "Oooohhhh," said Xavier, "I want this one," and he grabbed a devil puppet. "I want the puppy, mommy," Monica said. I told the children that they could pick out the puppets they wanted and mom and dad would be picking their puppets out as well. "Dad's gonna get a puppet?" screamed Xavier. "That's right," I responded, "everyone in the family is going to have their own puppets." I continued to speak as mother and father began to explore the puppets: "What I want you to do once you've chosen the puppets is to make up a story that has a beginning, a middle, and an end. It has to be a made-up story, not one like Cinderella (La Cenicienta) or Pinocchio. I'm going to give you about 30 minutes to make up your story and then when I come back in I want you to act out the story." Xavier asked me where I was going and I pointed to the one-way mirror, while telling him that I was going to the room behind the one-way mirror and would watch them make up their story, and then return to where they were when their story was ready.

When I got behind the observation mirror, I saw Tony sit back in his chair, apparently waiting for the others to pick the puppets they wanted. The more mother limited Xavier to one puppet, the more he wanted all the puppets. They argued about whether or not they could each have more than one puppet, until mother stopped insisting when Monica picked three puppets for herself. "Alright, alright," she told Xavier, "pick as many as you want, but be sure you leave some for your dad." Father leaned over and took two puppets and mother decided on a puppet as well.

Xavier initiated the story and argued with his mother over its direction. Father had little to contribute during this stage of the game, and seemed satisfied to take directions from his son and wife. Monica had very few demands or ideas. Mother included her in the story from time to time, but it was Xavier who dominated the process. After 20 minutes they finished the story, since mother was constantly watching the clock to make sure the task was completed in the assigned time. I reentered the room and told them I was very much looking forward to hearing their story. I instructed them to see me as the audience and act out their story for me. Xavier began . . .

SKUNK (Xavier): I'm a skunk, and everywhere I go I whiff out a bad smell and everybody runs away holding their nose. I got the baddest smell around. Nobody can mess with my smell. Pee-You. That's my name, Pee-You. And pee-you, too, to Mr. Fat Old Whale.

WHALE (mother): Well, I'm the whale and I'm very big and swim in the vast ocean. I'm the biggest fish in the sea, and other fish respect me because I'm very powerful and very wise. And by the way, I have a very nutritious diet of sea weeds. I don't like the trash that people throw out of their boats. I guess you'd call me a vegetarian whale.

PUPPY (Monica): That's good so you don't eat me. Whales don't like to eat puppies, only sea food, sea fish.

WIZARD (Xavier): I am the smartest not you, old fat whale. I am the wizard, not of Oz, but of Oooozzzze; I oooozzzze out smartness. I know things others don't. I know things about everything. Like I know that sharks are really friendly and they don't eat people unless people are using tanning lotion that smells good to them and then they eat them, but otherwise you leave them alone, don't you, Mr. Shark?

SHARK (father): I'm the mean shark.

PUPPY (Monica): Not the mean shark, daddy, you're nice—

SHARK (father): Okay, I'm the nice shark except sometimes people think I'm mean.

WIZARD (Xavier): Because people don't know anything—

SHARK (father): Yeah. People don't know the real me. (*Turning to me, father asks, "Should we be telling a story or what?" I respond, "Yes, tell me a story with a beginning, a middle, and an end."*)

SHARK (father): One day there were fishermen in the sea trying to catch me and I kept evading the spears they were throwing . . . and they even sent a guy down to the ocean in a jail, I mean a cage, and they tried to trick me by giving me a big fish to eat, and he was bleeding and stuff and smelled real good but I'm no dummy, I saw that it was a trick.

XAVIER: But dad, you're supposed to get caught so we can help you.

FATHER: Oh, that's right.

SHARK (father): One day though, I guess I had a headache or something because I wasn't thinking very well, and they sent down a really good-looking girl shark.

WHALE (mother): Don't you mean a good-looking whale?

SHARK (father): Sharks don't like whales, Fern, you know that.

MOTHER: Well that's what we agreed on.

FATHER: No, we didn't. You're supposed to help rescue me.

MONICA: Yeah, with me mommy.

MOTHER: Alright, go on then.

SHARK (father): So anyway, the girl shark was wearing lipstick and she had big earrings.

MONICA: Daddy, sharks don't wear earrings, silly.

XAVIER: Shut up stupid . . . it's part of the story.

MOTHER: Don't you call her names, Xavier.

XAVIER: Okay, okay, come on dad—

SHARK (father): So I finally went up to say "hello" and another cage fell on me and I was trapped and I didn't like it, so I hollered out for my friend the wizard.

WIZARD (Xavier): A fine mess you've gotten yourself into this time. I'm gonna help you out.

SHARK (father): I'm glad to hear that.

WIZARD (Xavier): Well, first, I've heard that sometimes dogs can scare away the fishermans and then we can steal their keys and get you out.

SHARK (father): That sounds like a great idea. Get me that yelpin' dog.

XAVIER: Come on, Monica, get the dog.

PUPPY (Monica): Ruf, ruf, ruf, ruf, ruf.

MOTHER: Louder honey, you want to scare those fishermen.

PUPPY (Monica): Ruf, ruf, ruf, ruf.

WIZARD (Xavier): I have another idea, Mr. Shark. I'm going to ask the biggest, fattest, strongest whale in the ocean to come and break your cage.

WHALE (mother): I'm the biggest and strongest. Let me at that cage. Where is it? (*Mother actually dives straight into the shark's body as father seems uncertain how to react. The kids are laughing as mother slams her fist into the shark's belly.*)

SHARK (father): Well as strong as you are, Whale-o, you're not strong enough to help me. I want out. Mr. Wiz, Mr. Wiz, what's your next idea?

WIZARD (Xavier): Don't worry. I got another idea. I have a friend who has the worst smell in the ocean. He'll get you out. Here he comes.

SKUNK (Xavier): Get ready one and all, here comes my powerful smell. When I woof it out everyone will be out of here in a hurry. Okay, here it comes. Get ready. Wwwooofff. Take that you mean guys. You can't keep my shark in your jail. Wow, those jail walls are melting. . . . Those fishermans are speeding away in their motor boats. . . . Pee-You is here to save the day. He cleared everyone out of the ocean and rescued the shark.

SHARK (father): Thank you, Mr. Wizard, for setting me free again.

MR. WIZARD (Xavier): You're thanking the wrong guy. Pee-You's the hero here. He knows just how to get rid of everyone. He's one powerful skunk. He did what no whale and no puppy could.

MONICA: Mom, my birdie didn't get to try to save the shark.

XAVIER: No bird can save the shark. You're too late.

MOTHER: Xavier, let her try. She wants to use her birdie.

XAVIER: Mom, the shark's already free.

MOTHER: The shark can go in his jail again.

XAVIER: Mom, how come she always has to get her way?

MOTHER: Because she's little. . . . Come on, Xavier, you're wasting time, she could have already done it already. (*Xavier settles into a chair disgusted, and Monica grabs her bird puppet.*)

MONICA: Xavey, what do I do?

XAVIER: I don't care.

SHARK (father): I'm in my cage again. Oh, no, what will I do? Mr. Wizard said there was one last-minute try before he brought in his secret weapon. Oh, yeah, a bird was going to fly here and pick the lock.

BIRD (Monica): Oh, yeah, here I come daddy. I'm coming to save you. I'm going to open the key. It's too hard. Oh, oh, I can't.

MOTHER: Xavier, come on, let's finish the story again.

SHARK (father): Now, let's see, Mr. Wizard said there was a secret weapon . . . someone who smelled really bad . . . someone who would clear out the place. (*Father turns to Xavier, "Come on Xavey, don't be such a jerk. Let's just do it again."*)

XAVIER: Okay, okay, and the skunk comes over and stinks the place up and everyone leaves and the jailhouse melts and the shark is set free.

WHALE (mother): Well, I hope you'll know not to get tricked again Mr. Shark.

SHARK (father): No way. No way I'm going back to jail. Hello to you, too, Mrs. Whale. What's for dinner anyway?

WHALE (mother): Oh, the usual, fish and veggies. Why don't you stop in for a while for dinner, if you have time that is.

SHARK (father): I got all the time in the world. I'm a free shark. I'll come to dinner but only if Mr. Skunk and Miss Puppy and Miss Birdie come too. They tried to help me out, and Mr. Skunk managed to set me free—

WHALE (mother): Everyone's welcome to dinner.

XAVIER: That means Mr. Wizard too. The end.

WHALE (mother): Well that's an abrupt ending.

THERAPIST: Is that the end of your story?

MOTHER: I guess so.

Ordinarily, I leave closure questions, such as titles and lessons, until after I have made some interventions within the context of the story. I was surprised to find myself rushing, and I may have been responding to what I perceived as either the family's urgency or my own.

THERAPIST: Mr. Shark, what is the title of your story?

SHARK (father): A title. Hmm. I guess, "Freedom Is Best."

THERAPIST: Who else has a title?

MOTHER: "Guess Who's Coming to Dinner."

THERAPIST: What about Xavier and Monica. What are your titles?

XAVIER: "The Stinker Hero."

MONICA: (*Giggles.*) "Daddy Come Home."

I then stopped for a few minutes to consider how to proceed.

Clinical Impressions

I was somewhat overwhelmed by the rich and varied meanings presented by the family story. The story reflected and exposed some of the most obvious and subtle problems in this family's functioning. At the same time, the story held some surprises and revelations.

As I watched the story unfold, I found the father's participation moving and unexpected. In the previous session his physical posture, tone of voice, and limited responses indicated a lack of involvement in and understanding of the family. On the surface, he seemed uninvolved and even a hostile and resistant participant. Mother seemed to be a paradox of control: She appeared both to make all the decisions and verbalize constant directives, and yet she was ineffectual and felt incompetent and frustrated.

In the first session Xavier was uncontrollable, making rigorous attempts to distract the therapist from a discussion with the rest of the family. In retrospect, his behavior seemed almost heroic in that it protected his father and his parents' marriage. At the time, Xavier seemed to want and need a great deal of attention from everyone, and settled for negative attention from his mother. Early clues to these problems were provided by puppet selection. Xavier chose both a skunk, whose smell drives others away, and a wizard, who might perform magic tricks or solve life's most elusive questions. Mother chose a whale, perhaps reflective of her concern with both her own and her child's weight, as well as her desire to dominate and exhibit strength. Father chose two animals that are generally viewed as threatening—a shark, which can kill, and a spider, which likewise presents a lethal hazard. Father's choices were particularly revealing given his passive behavior. Monica chose three puppets that seemed congruent with her personality: a puppy, a small bird, and a little girl with braids and a smile on her face.

The process of scripting the story was interesting to behold. Mother and Xavier argued vigorously, both jockeying for dominance and control of the story's content, direction, and resolution. These two family members contained most of the family's energy. They fought as one might expect a couple to fight and Xavier persevered and usually wore down his mother. Father seemed content to be told what to do and Monica sucked on her fingers while listening to the active discussion between her mother and brother. She asked for little and allowed mother to champion her cause.

Although Xavier had wanted the spider's sting to engage in combat with the skunk's smell, once I entered the room to listen to the story it evolved differently as father took a more active role. The story's theme was simple: Father was jailed in a cage and needed to be rescued, and Xavier was the only one with the wisdom and special ability to rescue him. Although the wizard encouraged and allowed the whale (mother) and the puppy (Monica) to take a stab at helping the shark, they failed. Xavier was the only one in a position to help and through the skunk's smell freed his father. Monica felt left out of the story and asked for equal time. Xavier was unreceptive to her request and became sullen as she was allowed to have some attention. He grudgingly participated at the very end by contributing a title to the story.

There were many references to food, eating, and weight. Mother constantly referred to strength and the power of size. She also made undisguised references to eating healthful, using the story as an opportunity to drive home her points about healthy eating habits. When mother (as the whale) attempted to "help" father (playing the shark), she chose to do so by violently lunging her puppet into his, with the result that she was unable to penetrate his armor (i.e., the jail bars). It appeared that her style of helping could be hurtful.

Xavier's choice of a skunk reflected an aspect of his presenting problem. His weight was causing some rejection from others. As per his mother's reports, Xavier was spending more and more time alone since his friends ridiculed him constantly. Mother said she had been hurt this way as a child and wished her parents had taken more of an interest in her when she needed their help. Obviously, she believed that the most helpful thing to do was to badger Xavier into changing his eating habits. Unfortunately, her way of helping was hurtful to Xavier. It also appeared that Xavier found some paradoxical power in keeping others away from him through gaining weight. One possibility for this could be that in the "control struggle" with his mother, he had chosen a territory that was clearly within his control. As he kept his mother engaged in a struggle to control his eating, he also helped his father. If mother had disengaged from the struggle with her son, it is possible she would eventually have had to face her distance from, and lack of contact with, her husband. Tony, it appeared, felt constricted and without freedom. He needed someone's help to become free and his son was successful in this regard.

Many of these observations and thoughts spun around in my head as I tried to decide how to proceed. I thought about the skunk's repelling ability, the puppy's willingness to help, the whale's bigness and meanness and sense of helplessness, and the imprisoned shark. Finally, I chose to focus on the shark, partly to validate and encourage the father's continued participation.

THERAPIST: Mr. Shark, You've made an amazing escape from the jail. Tell me, How does it feel to have so many people interested in helping you?

SHARK (father): Uh, I don't know. A little different.

THERAPIST: Tell me more, Mr. Shark.

SHARK (father): Usually people are afraid of me and don't give me much of a how do you do?

THERAPIST: You mean you find yourself overlooked sometimes?

SHARK (father): You could say that.

THERAPIST: What would you say?

SHARK (father): I'd say ignored.

THERAPIST: Tell the whale what it's like to be ignored.

SHARK (father): Well . . . (*avoiding eye contact with the whale puppet*) . . . sometimes I feel like my opinion don't count for nothing.

MOTHER: Well, Tony, that's because you never say how you feel.

THERAPIST: Mrs. Whale, can I talk with you for just a minute? (*Mother puts the whale back on her hand as the kids watch quietly.*) Mrs. Whale, you were one of those who tried to help. Can you do me a favor? Are you willing to listen to the shark for a minute or two?

MOTHER: Yes, but I had to respond to the statement about being ignored.

THERAPIST: Well, yes, I'm sure there is a lot you and the shark have been waiting to say to each other. But for now, I'm wondering if you're willing to listen to the shark for a minute or two?

MOTHER: Sure.

THERAPIST: Thank you, Mrs. Whale?

WHALE (mother): Sure, alright.

THERAPIST: (*Realizing it would be more fruitful to encourage a positive exchange between the parents, I change my line of questioning.*) Mr. Shark, we were talking about how it felt for you to have so many people try to help you out of your cage. Please tell the whale what it was like to have her try to help you?

SHARK (father): Well, it was nice that you made an effort . . . you tried.

WHALE (mother): Even though I didn't—

SHARK (father): Well, it's the thought that counts.

THERAPIST: And what thought would that be?

SHARK (father): (*Addressing the therapist*) Well, you know, that she tried.

THERAPIST: Tell Mrs. Whale, not me.

SHARK (father): That you tried—that's what's important.

THERAPIST: And her trying made you feel how?

SHARK (father): (*Looking at therapist*)

THERAPIST: Tell Mrs. Whale, not me.

SHARK (father): It felt good that you tried.

THERAPIST: And you, Mrs. Whale, how does it feel to be appreciated for your efforts?

WHALE (mother): Except I didn't succeed.

THERAPIST: Mr. Shark, tell her again.

SHARK (father): I appreciate your trying.

THERAPIST: And—(*Looking at mother*)

WHALE (mother): Thanks. I'm glad I tried to. I don't know what you were doing in the cage to start with. (*Laughter*)

THERAPIST: Mr. Shark, could you tell the puppy and the birdie what it was like for you that they helped?

SHARK (father): Well, Mr. Puppy, when you barked you scared me. I'm surprised you didn't scare all them fishermen away . . . I thought you sounded like a good watchdog. And that birdie, I mean you Birdie, were so good at picking the lock you almost got me out. Thanks a lot. Thanks for helping me out.

MONICA: Thanks daddy.

SHARK (father): You mean fearsome shark.

MONICA: Mr. Sharkman.

THERAPIST: And now tell the skunk and the wizard how you felt being helped by them.

SHARK (father): Well, you, Mr. Wizard, are some smart enchilada. You knew just what to do, and you hid your secret weapon, Mr. Pee-Wee (*Xavier interrupts, yelling, "Pee-You!"*) Mr. Pee-You, you hid him well until the last moment and then he came out and saved the day.

SKUNK (Xavier): Yeap, that's me, Super-Pee-You.

SHARK (father): Thank you so much for hanging in there until you knew I was free—

THERAPIST: Tell the skunk and the wizard how you felt that they didn't stop trying until they were sure you were free? (Mother later told me she perceived this statement as a condemnation of her not persisting until she succeeded in helping.)

SHARK (father): Well, Skunk, your friend Xavey is a really special kid. He's my secret weapon.

At this point I decided to stop and let everyone absorb what had just happened. This family had probably not had a calm exchange among all of them in quite a long time. In fact, they sat for a while in silence, fingering their puppets and giving each other brief smiles.

THERAPIST: It's time to stop for today. I want to thank you for the way in which all of you participated in creating this story with the puppets. I found your story interesting and I'm sure we'll all think about this experience and the story you told throughout the week. I'll look forward to seeing you next week.

Conclusion

This family had brought their son to therapy for his "weight problem." The child was indeed overweight and seemed to be experiencing some rejection from friends. Mother and son were engaged in a battle over his eating habits, while father and sister watched quietly. Xavier got most of the attention in the family; Monica was compliant and quiet, and thereby elicited her mother's protective and nurturing behaviors. Xavier's father, Tony, had withdrawn from the family, seeking a quiet and neutral corner. Tony had been raised in a family in which verbal arguments were rare, and thus felt disturbed by the constant fighting in his house. Fernanda, the mother, had been raised by "neglectful" parents, who had not paid sufficient attention to her and her problems, choosing instead to feed her when she expressed fear, worry, or sadness. Fernanda had been obese all her life and felt mortified that her son would experience the same pain that she had. In an effort to give him "enough" attention, she had become intrusive and obsessed with his eating. The mother and son's struggle over control of the latter's eating habits also helped distract the mother, so that she did not recognize that she and her spouse were growing apart.

The family's puppet story helped to illustrate how Xavier's weight was designed to get his mother's attention and keep her focused on him rather than his father. Xavier later revealed that before his mother used to pick on him, she picked on his father, who usually retreated promptly. Father was able to describe feeling caged, which explained why he allowed his son to help him out of his predicament. Father was appreciative of all the attention he received from his family in the story and the theme of being ignored was broached.

In the following sessions, the children wanted to repeat the same puppet story verbatim, but I noticed that Xavier was eager to get to the part when I talked to the puppets and had them tell each other how they felt. On one occasion, Xavier motioned for me to come back into the room after only 7 minutes of the family's getting together to discuss their story had passed. The family used the skunk hero, caged shark, helpful puppy and bird, and frustrated and helpless whale as metaphors that allowed them to discuss family issues. In particular, both father and Monica began to delight in sharing attention with mother and Xavier. Both parents reported that since the first puppet story, mother had quit harping on what Xavier ate, and often the father (as shark) would caution Xavier to eat only seafood. Xavier was clearly more receptive to his father's admonitions about what to eat and seemed to appreciate his father's attention. As Xavier became less obnoxious, Monica began mimicking some of his most outrageous behaviors, which elicited a less acute response from both her parents than these behaviors had vis-à-vis Xavier.

As mentioned earlier, not all families provide the richness in symbolism that these two cases illustrate. However, many more families than we might suspect are predisposed to "talk in code" through play and stories, which may seem thinly disguised and obvious manifestations of underlying issues. Nevertheless, the metaphor provides the often needed distance and security to pursue a kind of self-disclosure perhaps only possible in this once-removed way.

Some families need a little more coaxing; and on occasion, I will wait a little longer to initiate this technique, show families a videotape of this technique (*Family Puppet Interview*, 1981), or tell a puppet story myself. Rarely, all these techniques fail to elicit the family's participation, and I employ other techniques instead.

Family Art Therapy

The visual arts have always been of interest to therapists because they represent a tool that individuals can use to show their experience of their world. Oster and Gould (1987) begin their seminal book on the use of drawing in therapy by offering a "historical review" of drawing. They assert that drawings and other forms of art have been observed, even in primitive times through etchings and carvings, as symbols that could express feelings, record actions, communicate ideas, and reflect cultural and religious beliefs and practices.

Drawing, as well as other expressive arts, have been used effectively in education, physical rehabilitation, and psychotherapy. In the late 1800s drawings became significant to the field of psychoanalysis, because they were thought to reveal aspects of the unconscious mind. Thereafter, both the fields of psychiatry and psychology quickly made attempts to structure the use of drawings to assess intelligence and personality. Goodenough developed an intelligence test in the 1920s based solely on the scoring of drawings (Kaufman & Wohl, 1992). Focus on the use of drawings as projective instruments began in 1940 by Machover (Machover, 1949).

The field of art therapy has evolved within the context of a considerable discussion about the potential benefits of art to the therapeutic process. Some art therapists put the emphasis on art and some on therapy. At the moment, art therapy is recognized as a field in and of itself. Indeed, a plethora of books on the subject of art therapy have been written in the last two decades. Some books focus on children's drawings (Di Leo, 1970, 1973, 1983), while others focus on the use of drawings in the assessment and treatment of all age groups (Gravitz, 1967; Hammer, 1968; Oster & Gould, 1987), and recent works have explored the drawings of children from violent or incestuous families (Wohl & Kaufman, 1985; Kaufman & Wohl, 1992). Developmental studies (e.g., Burt, 1921; Kellogg, 1970) have documented 20 basic scribbles of young children, thereby providing a clinical understanding of the developmental and psychological aspects of children's drawings.

Art therapy as a separate discipline emerged from psychoanalytic theories, which hypothesized that symbols represent forgotten memories and can emerge through dreams or artwork. Initially, clients were asked to draw the symbols they had dreamed so that clinicians could deal directly with the images as opposed to distorted verbal translations of them. Therefore, art therapy was traditionally used as an adjunct to psychoanalysis. In the United States, Margaret Naumburg finds "expressive" therapy to be complementary to psychoanalytic therapy, because

> it permits [the] direct expression of dreams, fantasies, and other inner experiences that occur as pictures rather than words . . . , [because] pictured projections of unconscious material escape censorship more easily than do verbal expressions . . . , [because] the productions are durable and unchanging, [since] their content cannot be erased by forgetting and their authorship is hard to deny . . . , and, [because] the resolution of transference is made easier. (quoted in Ulman, 1975, pp. 4–5)

Naumburg (1966) encouraged the use of art as a way to elicit and interpret specific themes revealed in the art. Kramer (1971) believes the art process itself to be healing without the use of verbal reflection. Rhyne (1973) finds that the use of art in small groups encourages self-expression, self-perception, and positive group interactions.

Oster and Gould state that one of the main purposes of psychotherapy is to "broaden the individual's experience of expression and relating" (p. 9). Further, "creating a concrete object—that is, drawings—makes it easier to communicate with others than to verbally acknowledge personal feelings, especially if those feelings are frightening" (p. 10). They go on to document the many clinical uses of art, stating art can be used as a diagnostic tool, as a measure of cognitive maturation, and as a projective technique. Probably the most widely used projective techniques are the "House–Tree–Person" technique (Buck, 1978; Buck & Hammer, 1969); and, elaborating on the use of person drawings as projective indicators of personality, the "Draw-A-Family" technique (Hulse, 1951), the "Kinetic Family Drawing" technique (Burns & Kaufman, 1970, 1972), and, more recently, the "Kinetic House–Tree–Person Drawing" technique (Burns, 1987).

For the purposes of this book, additional information will be provided only on those art techniques developed for and used by families. As mentioned above, Hulse's technique instructed individuals to draw a family to provide valuable information about their perceptions of the family. Hulse's instructions were simply: "Draw a picture of your family." Oster and Gould (1987) stated: "The resulting drawings tend to reveal a person's attitude towards family members and his/her perception of family roles. Family relationships are often expressed by the relative size and placement of the figures and by substitutions or exaggerations of the family members. It is sometimes seen that the examinee will omit him/herself from the family drawing, which is usually a reflection of feelings of rejection" (p. 47). Burns and Hammer developed the Kinetic Family Drawing technique, a useful modification of the Draw-A-Family technique, which introduces action into family drawings through increasing the amount of qualitative and quantitative information in the drawings. The instructions for this technique are: "Draw a picture of you and your family doing something together."

Oster and Gould note that individuals can draw families engaged in a passive activity, to reflect, for instance, scenes from the dinner table; themselves situated near or far from other family members; and scenes in which siblings are omitted, as well as scenes that include or omit themselves. They can also use diverse proportions in their drawings, and show different facial expressions. They go on to say that the introduction of drawings into family sessions is an alternative way of observing family interactions, and providing them with a medium for sharing family perceptions.

Rubin (1978) notes that family dynamics are revealed in drawings through their content, symbols, quantity, size, execution, the placement of the objects and figures, and the process whereby they are composed. Oster and Gould encourage clinicians to use family drawings because the activity's novelty will help them to gain information; to clarify goals for future interventions; to disrupt maladaptive ways of communicating amongst family members; to explore alliances that may inhibit family functioning; to equalize age differences; to enhance relationships through joint drawings; and to aid the expression of feelings in a nonthreatening way. In addition, they suggest that clinicians discover much about the family by observing the drawing process:

> [The clinician can] observ[e] who leads or follows, who is assertive or passive, who is resistant, and so on. . . . Symbols used by individual family members often address such issues as what or who is important to them and how they relate to other family members. . . . Destructive tendencies toward family members may be observed during the drawings. . . . The amount of time taken by a family to complete a drawing also may be of importance. (p. 115)

Despite the amount of information available, Oster and Gould say "Interpretations of drawings are only made after the family has been seen long enough for the clinician to recognize consistent symbols, patterns in execution, and so on" (p. 116). Landgarten (1981), with a slightly different perception, cautions: "Interpretations definitely are not made initially, as they may be too premature and inaccurate or insulting to the family which might jeopardize any future therapeutic involvement" (p. 116).

Although the Draw-A-Family and the Kinetic Family Drawing techniques sought to enhance the clinician's and family's understanding of perceived roles and relationships, and attempted to increase expressive communication, it is Kwiatkowska who first proposed using art therapy within family treatment. Ulman and Dachinger (1975), describe Kwiatkowska's work as incorporating art therapy with a newly developed psychotherapeutic technique called "conjoint family therapy." Although Kwiatkowska likens family art therapy to group art therapy, she also describes it as unique because

> we deal with a group which is not merely linked by their general maladjustment or by a common symptom. The family has lived as a group for many years . . . they have developed their own interactional pattern and a whole underlinked system of defenses. They have formed subgroups within the family group, alliances of some members of the family against others, and developed their own patterns of thinking which have produced the special culture or climate of a given family. (Kwiatkowska, 1976, p. 114)

Kwiatkowska (1978) initially used art therapy with schizophrenic families and found that although the emphasis of therapy should always be placed on spontaneous self-expression, certain structured tasks are also fruitful. For example, she found the "Joint Scribble" technique, in which the family makes a joint picture out of a scribble after each family member has made a picture out of his or her own scribble, to be beneficial. Kwiatkowska (1976) distinguishes family art therapy from other techniques, in the following way:

Families are here engaged in an expressive activity simultaneously, something which is impossible in verbal communication. The informal situation, the indirectness of the communication in art therapy, lessens superego defenses and controls. The symbolic images express unconscious feelings and gradually help to uncover and clarify ambivalent and confused attitudes within the family, feelings which are often too intense to express in words. Thus, in some instances, the therapeutic process can be accelerated by the family art therapy program. (pp. 37–38)

She (1967) adds that a standardized 2-hour family art interview should be conducted as soon as possible by an art therapist and an observer (i.e., a mental health professional) who has been working with the family. Although the role of the "observer" is not fully defined, she provides a case example to illustrate how the observer can be a catalyst for change within the family's drawing. Kwiatkowska (1967) describes a case in which a mother's drawing showed herself and her husband sinking in quicksand. The art therapist wondered out loud how anyone would know their help was needed if the couple did not reach out for help. The mother drew a hand reaching up while the participant-observer drew a helicopter overhead with a hanging rope ladder. The father then drew two little figures on the helicopter with mother left behind, while the identified patient drew a one-legged figure stretched out between her father in the helicopter and her mother's hand sticking out of the mud. This was described as a turning point in the therapy.

The standardized procedure Kwiatkowska uses consists of having each family member draw a "picture" of the family after doing a free drawing, which is the activity that begins the session: an abstract family portrait (i.e., "what you feel" vs. "what everyone looks like"); a scribble; occasional spontaneous drawings; a portrait of a parent/offspring; and finally a free picture at the end of the session. Many aspects of the standardized interview have been suggested by patients themselves. Kwiatkowska (1975) asserts that the emphasis of family art therapy is always on spontaneous self-expression, although standardized procedures have been developed for a more accurate comparison of different families' responses.

Rubin (1978) includes three art tasks in her 2-hour family evaluation: first, an individual picture done from a scribble; second, a family portrait followed by sharing among family members; and, third, a joint mural on paper, which is taped to the wall. Landgarten (1981) suggests the use of "problem-solving" art tasks. For example, she instructs family members to draw their initials as large as they can, and then to find a picture in the initials by elaborating on them, to title their picture, and to share it with other family members. In addition, family members are asked to work on one piece of paper and use different colors from other family members, so individual contributions can be recognized. (Larger families are split into teams to draw.) Sobol (1982) recommends using two kinds of art assignments: conjoint drawing tasks that interrupt or intervene in hierarchical sequences or family coalitions and individual drawings that will help a particular family member express him/herself. She also suggests using certain tasks such as "Do a drawing to represent why you think you are here," or "Draw what you think the problem is," in the early stages of treatment. Other specific techniques are described below.

THE FAMILY ART THERAPY CRISIS INTERVENTION MODEL

This model, which Linesch (1993) developed based on her work with families in crisis at the Benjamin Rush Center in Los Angeles, includes art interventions designed to promote the following sequential goals: (1) a cognitive understanding of crisis dynamics (e.g., by asking people to draw the crisis events and include what happened the day or hour before they contacted mental health, and/or to draw their family before and after the crisis occurred); (2) the ability to identify and express crisis-related affect (e.g., by asking family members to choose pictures in magazines that describe how they feel about the crisis, and/or by asking family members to draw themselves as they feel inside and as they imagine they look to their family); (3) an exploration of previous coping mechanisms and a facilitation of adaptive coping strategies through problem solving (e.g., by asking family members to draw as a group how they coped with a similar situation in the past, by asking family members to choose pictures or draw images that describe different possible solutions, and/or by asking family members to represent how they are now and how they wish to be in the future); (4) anticipatory planning (e.g., by having family members choose magazine pictures that represent their worst family fears and/or by having them draw pictures that represent how they would cope); and (5) a summary of gains made during the intervention process (e.g., instructing family members to portray themselves at the beginning and end of treatment, and by reviewing the family's artwork, since it provides a graphic record of the treatment process). She goes on to say that the "process of creating the artwork, the content of the artwork, and the interchange stimulated by the art activity" are vital aspects of the intervention (p. 27). Linesch and colleagues offer specific case examples with a variety of different populations and a range of problems (Linesch, 1993). She finds that the "psychotherapeutically directed art process can uniquely and effectively meet the needs of families" (p. 155). Specifically, she believes that the art process "facilitated members' affective self-expression; encouraged genuine communication between family members; and helped empower family members to acknowledge, take responsibility for, and hopefully modify their roles within the family system" (p. 155).

THE SCRIBBLE TECHNIQUE

After each family member has developed a picture from his/her own scribble, the family is encouraged to make a "family scribble." One person makes a scribble and everyone tries to find pictorial suggestions in it. Then each paints on this picture in order to bring it to completion.

THE SQUIGGLE-DRAWING GAME

Developed by Winnicott (1971), this technique seeks to establish communication with the child's inner thoughts and feelings. The technique consists of asking family members to take turns making pictures out of the previous person's squiggle. The child is subsequently asked to select his/her favorite squiggle and make up a story about it. Claman (1993), in an adaptation of this technique, gives the following directions:

> Each of us will have a piece of paper and a pencil. I will draw a squiggle and you will make any kind of drawing you like out of it, then you'll make up a story about your drawing, and I will ask a few questions about it (your drawing and story). Then you will draw a squiggle which I will make a drawing out of, tell a story about it, and you can ask me questions about it. (p. 178)

This game is continued, Claman suggests, as long as it is "therapeutically productive and interactively enjoyable" (p. 179).

THE FREE DRAWING TECHNIQUE

"Free drawing" consists of asking each family member to draw a picture of whatever he/she wishes. Then each family member is asked to share his/her picture with the family. They can also be instructed to draw whatever they wish on a single sheet of paper as a group. When asking the family to do a free drawing, large easel paper is offered.

THE COLOR-YOUR-LIFE TECHNIQUE

This technique was originally developed for children by Kevin O'Connor (Schaefer & O'Connor, 1983) to teach them about the expression of affects, to gather information about their affective life, and to elicit intense feelings on the part of the child. The technique consists of therapists asking children to pair an affect with a particular color (e.g., red = anger, purple = rage, black = very sad, green = jealousy, yellow = happy), until each color is associated with a particular affect. O'Connor suggests that most children can manage about eight or nine pairings successfully. (I often make a color chart that lists the associated affects and colors so that children have a quick memory refresher.) Children are then given a piece of blank paper, and told that the paper is going to be "filled up with colors to show the feelings they have had in their lives" (p. 255). O'Connor suggests saying something like, "If you have been happy about half the time in your life then half of the paper should be yellow," to illustrate the therapist's expectations of the task (p. 255). Children can then complete the task in any way they wish, using squares, circles, lines, designs, boxes, and so forth. Since the overall purpose of this technique is to encourage the verbalization of feelings, therapists encourage active discussion throughout. When presenting this task to a family, each individual member should be told to make up a separate color chart and a separate drawing of his/her life experiences. Family members are then encouraged to show the finished product to each other, telling as much or as little about it as each wants, or, as may be appropriate, about their life experiences.

THE SERIAL DRAWING TECHNIQUE

John Allan (1988) describes "serial drawing" as a scenario in which drawings are done every week in front of the counselor. This way, the pictures can be analyzed over time, rather than simply viewing discrete products. Thus, a family who is asked to draw kinetic family drawings may reflect the conflict or harmony in current interpersonal relationships in an ongoing basis. This technique can work well with other forms of creative

expression such as sandplay, drama, painting, clay work, and
so on.

THE BLOB-AND-WET-PAPER TECHNIQUE

Blobs and dribbles are made on wet paper with inks, watercolors, or other water-soluble paints. Wet paper can then be crumpled and spread flat. Inkblots can be made by dropping colors on pages and folding them. Glue can be spread out to hold some of the crumpled papers in place, or glitter or sand can be sprinkled over the glue to add texture to the painting. Families can also experiment with making joint "paintings" using this technique. Often, family members report they are able to express themselves by use of these tactile techniques and feel relief after using them.

THE THREE WISHES TECHNIQUE

Family members are asked to draw three wishes. They then share and discuss these drawings among themselves. Issues such as the strength of the wishes, how the wishes might come true, what wishes could be traded or exchanged with others, and so forth, are discussed.

THE DRAW-SELF-AS-ANIMAL TECHNIQUE

Family members are asked to draw themselves as the animal they would most like to be. Choices are then explored whereby each individual explains his or her reasons for them, including the valued or desired traits of the chosen animal. Family members can be asked to say which animal among them they are most/least like, and with which animal they would most/least like to spend time with.

FAMILY SELF-PORTRAITS

Family members are asked to draw a picture of themselves and to then show their self-portraits to the group. As a variation on this activity, all pictures can be placed face down and individuals can choose a drawing from the pile, then give an "introduction" to the person whose drawing they have chosen. Family members can also be asked to draw a picture of the family member sitting to their right and then show the drawing to the rest of the group.

FAMILY ABSTRACTS

Family members are asked to make an abstract portrait of how they feel as specific issues, problems, or concerns are being discussed. Clinicians offering families this opportunity should provide an array of color pens, pencils, and pastels, always ensuring that there are enough to go around.

THE KINETIC FAMILY DRAWING TECHNIQUE

Another useful exercise (developed by Burns & Kaufman, 1970) is to ask family members to draw a picture of themselves and their families doing something together. The families then present their drawings to each other. Clinicians can stimulate insights by asking family members what they notice, what they find significant, what they are surprised by, and so on. While they do so, the clinician observes interactional styles, power and dominance issues, displays of inhibition or disinhibition, affective expressions, and other process–oriented information. In addition, the content and themes of drawings are documented. Important information can surface as a result of family drawings, such as in the case of Figure

5.1 below. With this family drawing, a 13-year-old Caucasian youngster expressed her family members' primary strengths and weaknesses: It showed that they could function well on an intellectual level, but were cut off from their feelings. This drawing of family members with missing bodies reflected several concerns. Malchiodi (1990) notes that several authors have observed bodies without lower halves in the drawings of sexually abused children (e.g., Kelley, 1984; Cohen & Phelps, 1985); however, a careful assessment of this family alleviated concern over abuse. In fact, the drawing of family members without lower halves was the child's way of showing a family with negligible affective expression. The fact that all family members are separated from one another by a frame indicates "lack of communication and feelings of isolation" (Di Leo, 1983, p. 72). In addition, Kaufman and Wohl (1992), note that the absence of the neck alerts us to the possibility that the youngster "may be having difficulty with bodily impulses and concerns"; further, the neck connects the head with the body and "signifies the modulation between thoughts and

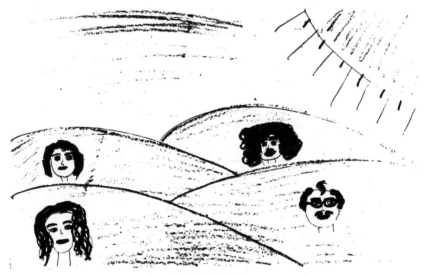

FIGURE 5.1.

drives" (p. 28). The 13-year-old had been referred for obesity and other self-injurious behaviors (cutting her arms with sharp objects). From exploring the drawing, it became clear that her eating and self-injury served as a way of coping with an emotionally barren environment. Her symptoms served to self-nurture, elicit familial attention, and block feelings of depersonalization.

With Figure 5.2, a lonely and unresponsive 14-year-old Caucasian boy attempted to communicate his sense of isolation. In this drawing his family is moving away from him, and toward an amusement park. He, in turn, is left behind. His perception, which was accurate, was that his parents were very bonded to his sisters, but were somehow unable to relate to a male child. The parents slowly revealed that their first-born child had died when he was 8 months old from a severe case

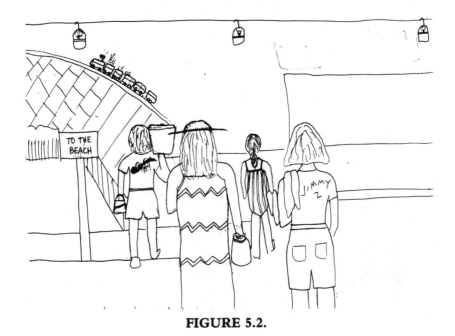

FIGURE 5.2.

of dehydration and they had been fearful their next son would suffer the same fate. Consequently, they had "kept their distance" from him and tried not to get overinvolved. When their daughters were born, they had felt less anxious about attachment and thus provided a nurturing environment for them. The youngster who made the drawing had felt "left out in the cold," and the family participated in long-term therapy to address their ambivalence about bonding with their son even at this late stage. Their attempts to include the boy were only marginally successful. Interestingly, he moved out of his home and married at the age of seventeen. He and his young wife sought therapy for "intimacy problems." At this time, therapy for this family member, was quite successful.

Figure 5.3 was drawn by a 12-year-old Caucasian boy named Danny, who was described as being "beyond parental control." Soon before coming in for therapy, he had been placed in a foster home, since his mother had felt unable to control his unruly behavior. Danny had been physically and sexually abused during his early childhood, and had lived with a physically ill mother intermittently. He had had a very unstable background, with numerous residences and schools. He was very unreceptive in treatment and resistant to verbal discourse. During the third session, I asked Danny to draw a picture of himself. His drawing was very compelling. There were many fascinating aspects to his self-portrait, which gave me much information about how he was feeling. The self-portrait seemed to reflect an internal conflict between his "good" and "bad" selves. The "bad" side was more defined. His hand looked like a conglomeration of clubs. He also had a "symbol of injury"* on his head and on his heart. With the

---

* Dr. Ann Burgess coined this phrase to define an idiosyncratic symbol which sometimes appears in the drawings of traumatized children. Children do not label these symbols; rather, clinicians deduce the meaning of these symbols by observing consistency, placement, size, and so on.

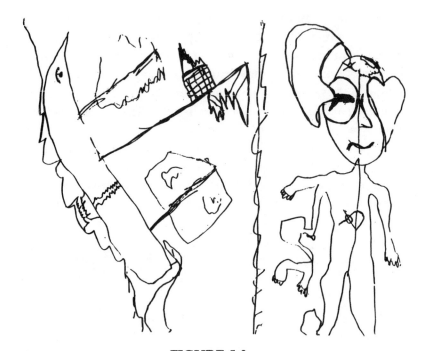

FIGURE 5.3.

drawing, Danny could communicate how vulnerable he felt by the size and the placement of his symbol. During one session, he drew a small head on top of a huge circle with an "X" that filled the entire page. This was done on the day that he learned his mother had missed yet another appointment with the school. For some reason, he had fantasized that his mother would come to the school and take him home with her.

The other half of his drawing was also of concern. The ship depicted here could not sail, since the sails were torn and shredded, and the keel was broken in half. The message seemed to be "I'm sinking." Danny's ability to express his true feelings in a more direct fashion was constricted by fears that no one would care or be of help. His experience to date had made him self-reliant, and think that his best defense was to fight and push others away, thereby giving the impression he didn't care about anything or anyone. The school had recommended that he attend therapy for his violent behavior, and thus his foster mother had started to bring him for sessions. After he made his self-portrait, I tried to elicit his impressions, but he was unresponsive. Because it was clear he was in distress and because I wanted to ensure environmental safety, I talked to Danny about meeting with his foster mother, and possibly sharing the drawing with her. "I think we have a lot to learn from your drawing," I told him, and asked him to think my suggestion over. The following week he acquiesced to my request that he show the drawing to the foster mother. Then I asked the foster mother a few questions and she responded as follows:

THERAPIST: What do you think of this boat?

FM: I think it's having a hard time.

THERAPIST: How so?

FM: Well . . . first of all, it's trying to sail uphill.

THERAPIST: That would certainly be hard.

FM: Yeah, and I don't know if there's much wind, but those sails aren't going to work too good.

THERAPIST: How so?

FM: Well, there's not much there . . . they won't be able to help the boat sail. . . . They're, how to say it, kind of useless, or used up, or something.

THERAPIST: What else do you notice?

FM: Well, the boat might be sinking.

THERAPIST: Why do you say that?

FM: Because it looks like it's broken on the bottom.

THERAPIST: Why would that be a problem?

FM: If the bottom's broke, the boat might not be able to stay afloat—

THERAPIST: Oh, oh.

FM: I hope the boat has a good radio on board.

THERAPIST: What else might help?

FM: Well . . . if there were some other sails folded up in storage.

THERAPIST: Good ideas, anything else?

FM: Well . . . I don't see the skipper, but I hope he's got a good first mate.

THERAPIST: So there are lots of ways to help this sinking ship.

FM: Yeah, if the skipper wanted to—

THERAPIST: So the skipper has to want to get the boat out of harm's way.

FM: In a matter of speaking—

THERAPIST: Danny, what do you think?

DANNY: I don't care.

THERAPIST: You don't care? About what? What was the question?

DANNY: I don't know and I don't care. . . . How long has she got to stay here with us?

THERAPIST: Well, I think she's looked at your drawing very carefully and had some interesting things to say about it . . . I think she can go wait outside anytime she's ready—

FM: Oh, I'll go outside now—

During the following weeks the foster mother told me that she had unconsciously called Danny "Skipper" a couple of times. She also told me that she had been very moved by his drawing and the dilemma it represented. I also was very concerned about his drawing and the symbolism of a "sinking ship." So much so, that I referred him for a psychiatric evaluation regarding suicidality and I constantly raised the issue of the ship with Danny, by talking to him about the many ways to salvage the situation and decrease the perceived harm. Although he seemed disinterested at first, he became more involved with the discussion when I offered him a model sailboat to construct in the therapy sessions. Suddenly, when the symbol became concrete, he spent considerable time discussing voyages, crews, the ship's maintenance and upkeep, and so on. As he carefully constructed his boat, his aggression seemed to dissipate a bit. His therapy continued for 2 years. During that time, he had two foster home moves before stabilizing in the home of a foster father while his mother continued to make little progress. It seemed inevitable that Danny would remain in foster care for a much longer period of time, as it turned out until majority. Obviously, the placement moves and the reality of mother's deterioration were monumental issues during his treatment, along with his victimizations, his longing for a parent figure, and problems with social interactions and impulsivity. His therapy had periods of resistance, multiple crises, and a short hospitalization for acute depression.

Figure 5.4 shows one of Danny's last drawings. This was the first drawing he made depicting a human being other than himself. Throughout the treatment, Danny had maintained his distance from me, being reluctant to accept my help. He had also had an ambivalent attachment to his foster father but recognized that he was trying hard to "stick" to him. In the drawing, Danny's symbol of injury (a barometer for feelings of vulnerability or despair) is barely detectable—it is the center of the flower being watered by the gardener. My interpretation of this drawing was very optimistic: Danny was finally absorbing the nurturing provided to him. There was hope for his continued growth and development. It was interesting that the gardener was a man. Perhaps the man represented the father he never knew, or his current foster father, and yet he wore a sailor's hat, which was reminiscent of his first foster mother, who had purchased herself and Danny sailor's hats shortly after the session in which his first drawing was explained.

Art therapy can be useful as an adjunct to other forms of therapy, or as a distinctive form of therapy, depending on the

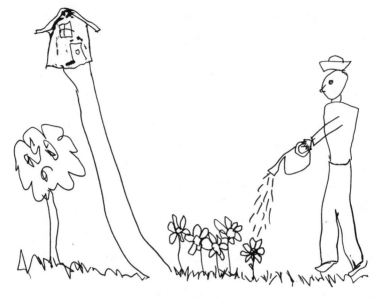

FIGURE 5.4.

clinician's training, experience, and comfort with this medium. Although most art therapy techniques have been used with individuals, there is ample room for using art therapy to engage families in useful and meaningful understanding and exchange or for understanding children's perceptions of family relationships. The use of art with families continues to be underemployed and research of its potential impact has been sparse; however, the gifted clinicians and art therapists referred to in this chapter have contributed greatly to our comprehension of the plausible utilizations of art with families.

The Mutual
Story-Telling Technique

Developed and described by Richard Gardner, the Mutual Story-Telling Technique (MSTT) shares similarities with the puppet interview (Gardner, 1971). The primary difference is that puppets are not used to tell the story. Instead, the child verbally reports an original story with a beginning, middle, and end. With this technique, "the therapist, on hearing a story, surmises its psychodynamic meaning, selects one or two important themes, and then creates a story of his own, using the same characters in a similar setting. . . . However, the therapist's story differs from that of the child in that he introduces healthier resolutions and maturer adaptations" (Gardner, 1993, p. 200).

Although widely accepted as a creative and useful technique, some therapists take issue with its potential (from a psychoanalytic standpoint) as a therapeutic, as opposed to a diagnostic, technique. These therapists tend to take issue, in general, with "directive" techniques, as the following statement implies: "The psychoanalytic concept of therapy relies on creating a therapeutic climate that promotes natural, evolving, moment-to-moment, spontaneous self-expression through play and verbalization with a *minimum* of structuring and interference by the therapist. The therapist's job is to help the patient expand on whatever the patient initiated, not to introduce anything new

. . . even when the child may be resisting" (Levenson & Herman, 1993, p. 227). These authors contend that clinicians must choose techniques that fit in with their theoretical belief systems. Hence, it is not surprising that a psychoanalytically trained therapist might take issue with most of the "directive" techniques.

With the MSTT, the clinician obviously interacts with children in a more active way, by listening to them, determining which character represents a child, and then identifying the story's primary theme and its resolution. More often than not, the child's ability to solve the conflicts presented in the story can be strengthened by providing alternative, perhaps healthier, strategies for resolution. This technique is helpful with many children because it works within the context of a familiar and primary medium of communication, the story. Because the child is asked to tell a story, instead of revealing information about the self directly, there is decreased resistance. Children will often reveal more information about themselves in this more comfortable mode. Indeed, their choice of themes, protagonists and antagonists, conflicts, and resolutions will reveal a great deal about their concerns, fears, and coping strategies.

Gardner engages the children in a playful manner by simulating an interview—that is, he sets up a situation where he pretends to be doing an interview show, and then audiotapes the interview. The interview is then labeled with the story's title, which the child provides, and is placed in a file. Hence, the child has clear evidence that this story-telling is something other children do routinely. The reason this technique is called "mutual" is that after children tell their story, clinicians tell the children a story as well. Clinicians prepare their stories by repeating back the children's stories as close to verbatim as they can recall. Children usually find this mystifying and may comment that it's their story that the clinician is telling. This repeating back of children's stories captures their attention. The clinical task is to recreate the story up to the point of the conflict, and then to introduce a conflict–resolution strategy that could be more functional. In this way, the clinician enters the child's metaphor to intervene within it. Because the child's symbols are used, the intervention can be understood on a deeper, metaphorical level.

CASE ILLUSTRATION 1

Marcus was an African-American 8-year-old boy, who was already in his third foster care placement. He had been removed from his biological mother when his elementary school teacher phoned the authorities regarding Marcus's violent behavior toward his peers. Marcus found many opportunities to injure his classmates and displayed violent outbursts of temper that were often unprovoked by any external incident. The teacher noted that Marcus's behavior was getting progressively worse both in frequency and intensity; hence, her concern about him as well as the other children grew. School personnel had made attempts to reach Marcus's mother to discuss the situation but she seemed unresponsive to their concerns. Indeed, she stated that if her child's behavior was a problem at school, it was not her problem. In addition, she had failed to keep numerous appointments with Marcus's teacher to discuss her son's academic progress, and had refused to open the door to the teacher when the latter had decided to make an unannounced home visit.

The incident that precipitated the school's call to the authorities was Marcus's fracturing of a younger child's nose when the child did not heed Marcus's directives to get out of his way. The yard assistant stated that when she reprimanded Marcus, he calmly said, "I don't care if I hurt him. Who asked him to get in my way?" This lack of empathy for others as well as his angry and provocative stance had become typical of Marcus. A psychological evaluation at school found him to be of normal intelligence, but functioning well below his potential. His academic performance had decreased sharply in the past year and a half prior to his entering therapy, and had started at approximately the same time as when Marcus's father had been murdered during a burglary of his store. Marcus's mother had found it difficult to cope with her husband's tragic death, and developed a strong dependency on alcohol to ease her pain.

The school felt that it was necessary to suspend Marcus from attending school, and when protective services interviewed the mother, they found her unable to care for her son in an appropriate manner. Efforts had been made to place Marcus with relatives but they declined, citing loyalty to his mother, who did not want her son placed with her relatives. (Mother later confided to me she was ashamed of her drinking and did not want her family to know of her condition.) Marcus was placed in a foster home where he injured the family pet. The foster family then requested his transfer, feeling he was potentially dangerous to their younger foster children. He had been in his second foster home less than 2 weeks when he set a small fire in his bedroom and was then sent to a specialized foster home where he was the only current resident. Throughout these events, he had constantly requested to see his mother, who had missed her appointments to see him. Marcus was referred for therapy as a result of his "conduct disorder" and potentially dangerous aggressive features.

Formulation of the Problem

Marcus's recent violent behavior was most likely directly linked to his father's violent death as well as his mother's inability to nurture him and reassure him after their shared tragedy. The mother's alcohol use most likely rendered her a sporadic and ineffectual caretaker. Marcus's mother seemed overwhelmed by her loss and did not seem currently capable of providing for her own care, let alone her young child's care. She had reportedly been unresponsive to school requests for meetings to discuss her son's problem behaviors. Marcus was probably aware of his mother's alcohol use, her impaired functioning, and her ambivalent feelings toward him since his father's death. I decided it would be important to contact the mother promptly to assess her functioning, and to determine if any services were being provided to her, the possibility of reunification, and her availability to cooperate and participate with her son's therapy.

The First Session

Marcus was the most overtly hostile and provocative child I had ever seen. His primary stance was to be on the attack: He called me names, threw toys against the wall, responded to specific questions with the use of profanity, and generally maintained a high level of intensity, which elicited a great deal of negative attention. He laughed as I attempted to review the office "rules," and he spit on me when I told him that I wouldn't let him hurt me or hurt himself. He ran from one end of the room to the other kicking toys and throwing things off the shelves. "This is not a good place for you to be," I stated, "Come with me."

I walked upstairs to another room that was available for children who found the smaller playroom too constricting. This room was large, sparsely furnished, and with very little toys or stimulation. The only objects in the room were a large couch, a few big pillows, a large chalkboard, and a Bobo. "You're not putting me in any box," he yelled as he followed me, reluctantly stomping his feet as he walked. "No, I'm not putting you in any box . . . we're going to a bigger room." When he got the Bobo, he immediately wrestled it to the ground, kicked it, fought with it, and got a tremendous amount of energy out of his system. He looked at me and said, "I can do what I want. I can kick him; I can make him bleed; I can punch his lights out." "Yes, you can," I stated, "because he's a toy, not a person." "I could even if it was a person." "You could," I said, "but it's not a good idea. You get into trouble and you hurt someone else." "I don't care," he said, hitting the Bobo again. "I understand you don't care right now, but it's not good to hit others because you will get into trouble." He did not respond verbally but seemed to calm down a little as he wandered around the room. He went to the large chalkboard and began to draw a poster of Bart Simpson. He was a skilled artist, and his picture of Bart was almost an exact likeness. "That looks exactly like Bart Simpson," I said. "I know," he said, "I'm a good drawer." "Yes, you are," I repeated, and I saw a glimmer of a smile. I put a cloud over Bart's head and without saying anything he wrote inside it, "I'll kick your ass."

On our way downstairs, Marcus pushed a poster on the wall so that it was crooked. It was his way of showing that he would still give me trouble even though we had shared a calm moment at the chalkboard. Before he left, I asked about the box: "What did you mean when you asked me about the box?"

"That other jerk stuck me in a box."

"What other jerk?"

"Dr. Pelts."

"What do you mean a box?"

"Nobody's doing that to me again."

"I don't have any boxes," I said, "don't worry about that!"

"You're a girl; you can't stick me in a box anyway." He ran out the door and the worker who had driven him to the session followed behind him in a panic. This first session had been tough. This child was in a great deal of pain and seemed very fearful of not being in control.

Early Sessions

The following four or five sessions duplicated the first session. Marcus set up rituals for himself that were predictable. He went directly to the large room, hit and hit the Bobo relentlessly, and then went to the chalkboard. Not much was said during any of this. Marcus drew cartoonlike pictures, mostly of Bart Simpson, apparently proud of his ability to draw. A couple of times I asked him to draw a picture of Bart's mom and dad, and he resisted the idea. "Maybe someday you will," I said. I wanted to address the issue of his mother and father. To date, he had refused to answer any formal questions regarding his mother, except to say "I don't know," or "I don't care."

I called the caseworker to ask about the psychologist who had seen Marcus once or twice before he was referred to me.

She gave me Dr. Pelts's telephone number and indicated that Dr. Pelts had suggested the child be placed in a secure residential facility. When I called Dr. Pelts, he immediately said there was very little information he could provide since he had only seen Marcus once. I asked how the session had gone. Dr. Pelts related that the child had been out of control, and that he had placed him inside a toy chest and sat on top of it to keep him confined for a period of time. I was aghast and said as much. Dr. Pelts then asked what my qualifications and training were and suggested I become better informed about working with children with obvious serious emotional problems before I proposed to work with Marcus. He seemed defensive and hostile as he announced, "That's all I have to say on the matter."

The next time I saw Marcus I told him I had talked to Dr. Pelts. He looked at me with wide eyes as I said, "It was wrong of him to put you in a box and not let you out. Nobody would like being held inside a box." "He's a jerk . . . I hate him," Marcus responded, and I said, "Putting you in a box was a jerky thing to do." He became quiet and drew some more.

I felt some urgency to create an environment where Marcus could begin to open up and thereby accept some of the support and help I could provide. At the same time, I had to respect his defensive posture. It was all he had to count on. I continued to try to make contact with his mother, who would not return my phone calls. I asked the people at child protective services if they were providing other services to her, and they said they were making weekly visits and transporting her to AA meetings; they were not too optimistic about her progress. They had approached her about visiting Marcus and she had responded by crying and saying that Marcus was better off without her. She had come to realize that she was not able to care for her son. The worker said mother felt ashamed and guilty about falling apart. On the positive side, perhaps the mother's realization that she was not functioning represented some type of progress. I asked for her address so that I might drop by her house in the evening sometime.

I decided that it might help the progress of the therapy to ask Marcus to tell me a story. He had been reluctant about answering questions directly, and at one point when I asked him what else he did well, in addition to drawing, he had said, "I tell good stories." At that time, he had refused to tell me one and I had said, "Maybe some day you'll want to." "How about telling me a story?", I asked, "I remember you said you told good stories." "What about?", he asked. "Anything you want . . . just make up a story with a beginning, a middle, and an end. Then later, maybe I'll tell you a story." He sat on a chair with the chalk in his fingers and told me the following story.

"There was a big house on a farm: not a city. They didn't grow animals there that they killed. They only grew vegetables to eat and the lady liked to grow flowers. The flowers were all different colors: black, green, red, yellow. She liked them all. She took care of them and gave them vitamins to grow bigger. Then one day a big bald dude came to the house with a big hose and a big long knife. He told her he was going to water the plants but then he took out his big knife and chopped all the flowers out. The lady cried and cried and never looked at her garden again. The end."

"What's the name of your story?" I asked. He did not like the question and firmly stated, "It has no name. It's just a story." "OK, here goes my story," I replied:

"Once upon a time there was a big blue house in a farm, not a city. No animals were grown or killed on the farm. The people grew vegetables to eat and the lady of the house liked flowers and grew lots of them of many different colors: black, green, red, yellow, orange. (*Marcus interrupts now and says, "Not orange, I hate orange." I correct myself.*) The lady liked all her flowers and took good care of them, and watered them and gave them vitamins so that they grew big and beautiful.

"Then one day a big, bald dude came to the house with a big hose and a long knife. He told the lady he would water her flowers but really he went over to the garden and chopped all the flowers down. The lady was very, very sad about her flowers and cried and cried and cried.

"Then one sunny morning something happened. The lady went and washed her face and, seeing how sunny it was, she peeked out the window at her garden. She hadn't looked at it in a long time because each time she did she would cry from sadness at having lost her flowers. She looked over and opened her mouth with surprise. She rushed to the closet, grabbed her shoes, all the while thinking about what she had just seen. She ran down the stairs, not believing her eyes, and she opened the door and ran around back to her garden. She was scared she hadn't really seen what she thought she had, after all, she was looking from the window upstairs and maybe her eyes had played a trick on her.

"As she got close, she saw her eyes had not played a trick on her. It was true. There they were. Little tiny, tiny, green blades peeking out. The cut flowers had been cleared away by someone and the garden was almost the way it was at the beginning: full of promise. She ran back in the house and asked the cook what had happened. 'Well,' the cook said slowly, 'I just felt so bad about what happened, and I thought maybe I could get the garden to grow again. I was going to tell you soon.' The lady hugged the cook and thanked her from the bottom of her heart. 'I can't wait to see my flowers grow again. Thank you for stepping in when my sadness wouldn't let me care for them.' She gathered up her old gardening gloves and vitamins and ran to her garden to care for the new flowers. The end."

"You know what the name of my story is?" I asked.

"It doesn't have a name. I don't want to know."

"Okay, if you ever change your mind you can ask me."

"That sounded like my story," he stated.

"Yeah, it sure did."

"I made that story up."

"Yeah, you sure did."

"My story was different than yours."

"Yeah, a little bit different."

"Mine was better."

"You thought your story was better than mine?"

"Yeah . . . it was."

"And my story was different than yours, in some ways, not all ways, just some ways."

"Can I go now?"

"Yeah."

"I wonder what your mom would think of your story."

"She wouldn't like it."

"It's hard to say. Maybe she would. Maybe someday you can tell her your story."

"I'm going," he said, and ran down the stairs and bolted out the door with the worker gathering her papers as she rushed behind him.

Commentary

Marcus's story exemplified his preoccupation with his mother and his own feelings of abandonment. In his story, everything is fine until a threatening male arrives with a hose and a knife. The mother is fooled by the man's offer to water her garden and allows him to get near it, which he then destroys. As a result, mother is devastated by her loss and doesn't want to look at her garden in order to avoid her pain. The garden most likely represents the life of both Marcus and his father. Father's life is taken in a violent way, and although mother loves Marcus, she becomes unable to invest emotional energy into his growth because of her sadness. Marcus also serves as a visible reminder of his father and mother cannot bear to have him near her.

In my story, I did not deny the events that had occurred in Marcus's life. A burglar had indeed entered the sanctity of Marcus's peaceful environment and murdered his father. Marcus's focus in his story was on his mother's abandonment after his father's death, although his father's death was also prominently featured. In my story, I also offered the idea that mother would be grieving for a period of time and that someone else might need to care for the garden until she was ready to resume her duties. I assigned the cook, a nurturing figure, the role of alternative caretaker. Unbeknownst to mother, the cook nurtures the garden and brings it back to life. Hence, when mother is able to peek out her window, she catches sight of new life in the garden, and rather than being saddened by it, she is filled with hope and anticipation.

After telling my story, I felt that I had been overly optimistic. While it was true that Marcus was being looked after by an alternative caretaker and that mother was in a state of paralyzing grief, it was unclear whether she was processing her grief or was stuck in it. In other words, I did not know if she was able to process the various grief stages and begin to feel motivated about the future. I decided to pursue collateral contacts with both the foster family and with Marcus's mother, who had to date been unresponsive to child protective services.

Contact with the Foster Family

Marcus had been in the specialized foster home since the time when he entered treatment, which amounted to 4 months. He was the only child in the foster home and, consequently, received all the attention he could tolerate. Initially, he elicited negative attention by breaking things, using foul language, and generally being provocative. When he realized that his foster parents would not hit him and didn't ask for his removal to another foster home, his behavior eased up a bit. He was still volatile, and his foster parents were baffled by his sporadic violent outbursts.

The foster parents were African-American and attended the same church services that Marcus and his mother had attended together. Marcus seemed both calm and sad after church services, and the parents believed he was deriving benefits from the regular exposure to familiar religious teachings.

I made contact with them during the first month of treatment. When we met, they were cooperative and interested in Marcus and how to be of help. I saw them very much as part of the treatment team and maintained contact with them on a weekly basis. I gave them forms to fill out about Marcus's behavior and any questions they had, and each week Marcus brought a form and handed it to me. The first time he had refused to give it to me without reading it first. I told him that would be fine, and, as a matter of fact, I would suggest to his foster parents that they fill out the sheet together so that there wouldn't be any secrets from Marcus. Marcus was fond of filling the sheets out and reminded his foster parents of all his troublemaking, just as they reminded him of all the positive things he had done.

The foster parents reported that on occasion Marcus became visibly distressed and asked for his mother. He expressed concern that without him she might die. At the same time, he said he would not care if she did die, thereby exhibiting his obvious ambivalence toward her.

Contact with Marcus's Mother

I asked the child protective services worker, Mrs. Chou, for the phone number of Marcus's mother. Mrs. Chou informed me that the mother's phone had been disconnected and gave me a street address. I went over at about 11 A.M. the next day and persisted at the door for about 15 minutes. Finally the door opened and Marcus's mother, Sonya, greeted me. She was very reluctant to allow me entry and asked that I return later in the day. I decided to make every effort to visit with her at the present time, and finally she acquiesced. She was drinking as we spoke, and it was unclear to me how much information would be processed or retained. My task was to assess the mother's interest in her son and the likelihood of her wanting to pursue a reunification with him.

I began by telling her what I knew about her situation. I reviewed the facts as I knew them as well as my understanding that she was attending AA meetings, although irregularly. I told her that since I began working with her child I was in contact with Mrs. Chou, who would give me an update regarding her progress. When I spoke about Marcus, mother became more attentive. She asked how he was, whether he was doing well in school, and whether he was being a "good boy." I responded that Marcus had both been through the same shock and trauma she had and thus was having a difficult time. Mother volunteered that it was different for Marcus in that he would soon forget his father since he was so young. "For me it's different," she went on, "It's as if my life has stopped also." I took the opportunity to make the following statement: "It is different for you and for Marcus. You lost your husband, and, believe me, I know how much that hurts you. Marcus, on the other hand, lost his father and his mother."

She stood up and walked to the counter to refill her drink. "He hasn't lost me . . . I'm still here," she said. "As far as he's concerned," I added, "he's lost you. He doesn't see you, talk to you, and sometimes wonders if you're dead or alive." "He's better off without me, I'm no good for him, I can't even give him what he needs most—his daddy," she said gruffly. "Not really," I responded, "Marcus loves you and misses you very much. You have both been through a tremendous loss and are hurting. You could be helping each other." "I can't help anyone right now" was her response. I could tell our meeting was coming to an end as mother's eyes were now barely open. "Your son needs you and has already lost one parent, " I said. "Please imagine what it would be like to lose both parents at the same time." I asked her if it would be alright if I came back to talk to her some more, and added, "What would be a good time to come so that we can talk together when you're sober?" Mother opened the door for me and said, "About 6 in the morning is good." I usually made early morning visits.

I came back four more times and mother asked about Marcus each time. I repeated my concerns over his experience of loss, and, finally, I told her that I had been coming to see her to find out if there was any interest on her part in becoming a mother to Marcus again. She insisted that he was better off without her, and I insisted that Marcus needed his mother and that until he had his mother nearby, he wouldn't be able to deal with his father's death. Finally, I told Marcus's mother that her allowing me in the door over the past month signified that there was a part of her that very much wanted to make contact with her son. I then told her that I wanted her to come to a family session with Marcus the following week. I added that I would make the appointment early in the morning so that she could attend it sober, and that I would make arrangements for Marcus to be excused from school so he could come in the morning. I told her it was time for Marcus to see that his mother was alive, and it was time for her to see her young son's face for herself. I stated that I would not tell Marcus she was coming so that he would not be disappointed if she did not show up. I also told her I was aware that there was a part of her that was ready to reconnect with Marcus and be his mother, and a part that wasn't ready to commit to life and her son. "I'm betting," I added, "that the part of you ready to be Marcus's mother will win out and attend the meeting."

I was reticent to tell Marcus that his mother would attend the session and then have him experience grave disappointment if she didn't show up. I opted instead to quickly prepare him to see his mom should she show up. I was nervous about whether Marcus's mother would show up or not show up. Twenty minutes into the session the secretary called my office to tell me the mother was downstairs. I hung up and looked at Marcus. "Marcus, your mother is downstairs," I said. He froze. "I invited her to come here today, but I didn't tell you sooner in case she didn't make it." "I'll wait here. Go get her," he instructed. "Okay, we'll be right back." Marcus must have needed the time to gain his composure—his excitement was barely contained and yet I could see his hesitation as well.

Marcus's mother looked as nice as I had ever seen her look. She had obviously taken care to look presentable to her young son. Her face looked freshly scrubbed, and she wore dark sunglasses, which I'm sure were meant to conceal bloodshot eyes. "Is he here?" she asked. "Yes, he asked me to come and escort you upstairs." "Does he want to see me?" "He didn't know you might come so he seems excited and surprised," I replied. When I walked in, Marcus was sitting in a chair. When he saw his mother, he bolted out of the chair and ran over to her, putting his arms around her waist. Neither of them spoke. They stood embracing each other for the longest time.

Mother finally broke the silence by saying, "Let me look at you," and she motioned him to direct his face upward. "Such a sweet boy." Marcus hugged her again and mother walked him over to the couch. They sat together, holding each other and crying softly for a very long time. They looked as if they were close to sleeping, so I interrupted with, "Marcus, I thought perhaps you could tell your mother the story about the garden." He reoriented himself to the room and my interruption. "I don't wanna." "How about if I tell the story?" I replied. "I don't wanna." Mother intervened, "I like to hear stories, go ahead and tell me your story Marcus." Marcus said, "Remember when I would tell dad stories and he would laugh?" "Yes," mother said, "I remember how you could make him laugh." "Tell me the story." Marcus repeated the story about the garden almost exactly the same as he had told it the first time. I added, "Marcus, tell your mom the story I told you." Marcus said, "Her story is the same as mine except in hers a cook takes care of the garden until the mother is finished being sad." I elaborated by repeating my story (I had documented both Marcus's and my stories, so I read them the story).

Mother seemed to understand the meaning of my story. "How about you? Do you want to tell Marcus your story?" I asked mother. She responded quietly,

"In my story the mother has been sick for a long, long time and hasn't even been able to look out the window at her garden. But in my story the mother is very, very lucky because she has people who are willing to help her, and slowly, very slowly, she begins to feel better, and she decides to take one day at a time and let God help her because, Marcus, God never gives us any more than we can handle. Eventually, the lady can take good care of her flowers because she's learned how to take care of herself, but it takes a long time, Marcus, because it's not easy to take care of yourself."

They held each other for the last 5 minutes of the session, and then I said the time was up and Marcus would have to go back to school. He protested loudly and mother said, "I will see you again soon. I can even come back here and see you, or I'll come see you in your foster home." Marcus smiled broadly as we set the next appointment.

Commentary

Following this session, Marcus and his mother met together in my office for about ten more sessions. In addition, mother visited him in his foster home once a week or every other week. Child protective services reported a vast improvement. Mother was getting herself to AA meetings two or three times a week and had secured a part-time job as a sales clerk. She had also entered individual counseling at a nearby mental health clinic and was in a bereavement group that was available for individuals who had been victims (or who were family of victims) of random violence. At this point, she was definite about working toward family reunification, and she was responsive to all suggestions.

This mother had been a functional and attentive mother and a devoted wife prior to her husband's tragic death. She had then become temporarily incapacitated from grief and alcohol abuse, but eventually made a decision to come back to her son and be the mother he needed. In the process she had committed herself to living without her husband. The sessions between mother and Marcus were not always easy. Marcus had a lot of anger to express and it appeared he was testing to make sure mother would be able to handle whatever he dished out without leaving him again.

Marcus had also grown attached to both of his foster parents, and although he was happy to be involved in a plan to return home, he was unhappy to leave his foster family. The foster parents were characteristically helpful in this transition. They offered to babysit for mom when she was busy or to invite them both to go out together from time to time. Mother did not have any jealous feelings about Marcus's affection toward them. Rather, she was grateful that they had been willing and able to care for him when she could not.

The reunification process took 6 months. During that time, there was a gradual increase of supervised and, later, unsupervised visits with mother. Mother made a remarkable and realistic recovery, aware that she would need to surround herself with a strong support system from now on. She was clear that her self-imposed isolation after her husband's death contributed to her dependence on alcohol, and she was determined to surround herself with friends, many of whom she had met at AA meetings, and her AA sponsor, a mature woman of color who had also endured a violent tragedy to her husband and enjoyed becoming a grandmother figure to Marcus.

Conclusion

The Mutual Story-Telling Technique was an effective strategy with this family. The story the child told contained a theme that could be conveyed to the mother and offer her a way to understand what had happened after her husband's death. Marcus had been unable to express his feelings verbally at first. He was most effective in showing his distress through behavior. But through using the story as a vehicle, with its metaphor of an unattended garden, he could talk about both the horror of his father's violent death and his feelings of abandonment from mother. Luckily, my intuition about mother was correct. I would have had to alter my story if mother was unresponsive to child protective service interventions as well as my own. Because mother had established a warm and positive contact with the child prior to the traumatic incident, I anticipated that the bond could be reestablished.

I made several provocative statements to mother when I first met with her. Mother later remarked to me that it particularly made her angry to hear me say that Marcus had lost both his father and mother while she had only lost her husband. Her anger against the concept that she was dead for her son was a motivating force that enabled her to fight back. In fact, her initial commitment was to live only for her child; eventually she was motivated to live for herself as well. Once her commitment was made, Marcus's mother was relentless in the focused way she approached her goal of reunifying with her son.

CASE ILLUSTRATION 2

Mandy was a 6-year-old Hispanic child who had gradually developed phobic behaviors that concerned her parents, Lupe and Muriel. Both parents were acculturated and preferred to speak in English. Lupe and Muriel attended the first session and related that Mandy had been a very "easy" child since birth. Lupe described her pregnancy as a "joyful and serene" time with basically no complications. She had had morning sickness for about 2 months of the pregnancy and virtually no discomfort thereafter. She said both Muriel and she had planned the pregnancy, thereby making Mandy "one of the most wanted children on this earth." Both parents were present at the delivery, which lasted about 4 hours. Muriel remarked, "even during her birth Mandy was a good kid . . . she really came quickly and without too much discomfort." Lupe agreed that the childbirth had been relatively pain free compared to what she had expected; her mother had always told her that childbirth was God's punishment to women.

Both parents described Mandy as delightful, carefree, sensitive, and full of joy. They had never explicitly described their homosexuality to her, but they had always demonstrated a loving intimacy in front of her free of shame. "At the same time," Lupe added, "we were both raised Catholic and we have a high sense of morality. . . . We have never been inappropriate in front of Mandy, and we keep our private life private."

Muriel related that in the last 6 months Mandy had changed. She had become clingy, introspective, and quiet. It was as if her usual spontaneity and joy were stifled somehow. Muriel said: "Before we could always count on Mandy for a good laugh. . . . She just says some of the funniest things. . . . She'd always be up for going on a drive, or a walk. . . . Lately it's almost as though she mopes around the house, and she doesn't seem as free or playful as she was before." When I asked the parents whether any particular things had happened in the last few months that could explain this change, Muriel commented that her father had died and that they had all attended his funeral. "We felt very guilty about that," she added, "like we should not have exposed her to a dead body . . . but the service was very low key; there was a closed casket, and our parish priest did the service. . . . Mandy has known him since she was a baby and she knows the church pretty well. We can't figure out what might have upset her but we think it may have to do with that." When I asked them how close Mandy had been to Muriel's dad, Lupe said softly, "He never accepted our relationship and although he was Mandy's grandfather he never paid any real attention to her. I'm sorry to say that he wasn't that close to her." Muriel added, "That's what's confusing to us . . . why his death would have troubled her. . . . He never came to visit us, for example; I would have to go over there if I wanted to see him."

I asked for other relevant information. The only other information that caught my attention was that Mandy had started school approximately 7 months prior to this session. When I asked how her first-grade experience was going, Lupe said that Mandy loved her school, loved her teacher, and that most of the children in the first grade had been her companions in kindergarten and thus were familiar to her. Lupe reported that she had a number of good friends in the class. Her best friends were older neighborhood children, Martin, a 9-year-old boy, and Stephanie, his 7-year-old sister. In addition, there was a set of twins across the street, Lois and Lana, who were 10 years old. Lupe and Muriel described their neighborhood as "friendly" and "easygoing." Muriel said, "Once a year we have a block party and everyone participates. We usually stay out on the street until about 3 A.M. We don't get much traffic on our street." Lupe added that most of their neighbors knew them and liked them, and they felt the same way. She said, "The only controversy in the neighborhood is a guy who doesn't keep his yard clean and stays to himself. He got real mad when we got a petition going to ask him to clear his yard of the junk."

Lupe and Muriel were both in their early 30s. Lupe was from Costa Rica but had lived most of her life in this country. She had a good relationship with her family, although she could not visit them with any regularity. Lupe stated, "Thank God, both my parents are active grandparents to Mandy, and they have visited once a year to spoil their granddaughter." Muriel, originally from Panama, stated that her family relationships were more conflictual than those of Lupe. Her father had been very distant with her and her siblings. Muriel did get along famously with her brother Scott, who, in fact, had donated the sperm for Mandy's conception. Scott also had a stable and loving homosexual relationship and Scott and his lover were affectionate uncles to Mandy. Muriel had a more strained relationship with her sister Rose, and thus had less frequent and warm contact with her. Muriel had not spoken to her mother since she was about 15 years old. At that time, Muriel's mother had left her children and husband and moved to another state. Scott had maintained enough contact so that he knew her current whereabouts but the relationship between Muriel and her mother had never been reestablished.

The First Session

Mandy was a petite and friendly 6-year-old, who shook my hand, insisted on speaking in English, and followed me into the playroom in a very trusting manner. Her parents had told her that I was a counselor who worked with children and helped them when they had any problems. I showed Mandy around the playroom, and she rapidly engaged in play with the dollhouse, making an orderly living room, kitchen, bedroom, and child's room with all the furniture. "Where are the family that live here?", she asked. I reached over for the miniature dolls and she put a little girl in the bedroom along with a puppy dog. "That little girl has a puppy dog. Do you?", I asked. "No," she responded, "but I would want a big dog who could watch over me." She then picked up two female dolls and placed them in the bedroom, one in bed and the other sitting near a vanity mirror. "They are going to sleep pretty soon," she said. She had the female doll at the vanity pretend to comb her hair, counting "55, 58, all done. . . ." The two female dolls then went to sleep as she covered them with a Kleenex. Mandy remarked, "This house don't got a roof." "That's right," I said, "No roof on this house." "Oh, oh, oh, no . . . they're in trouble now."

"What will happen to them?"
"They will catch cold."
"And then what?"
"Catch a cold?"
"Oh, they will catch a cold."
"They will, they will . . ."

"And then what will happen?" Mandy abruptly left the dollhouse and didn't respond to my question. She noticed the paper and pencils and asked if she could draw. She made a series of circles on a page, coloring each one a different color. After that she asked if she could color in one of the coloring books and she did that for the rest of the session. Before it was time to stop, she looked at me and asked me, "What other kids come here?"

"Lots of other kids," I said.

"Like who?"

"Boys and girls."

"How old are they?"

"Oh, your age, younger and older too."

"Do they play with the dollhouse?"

"Some of them do."

"Will they play with the dollhouse and wreck it?"

"Well, they may move things around."

"Don't let them, Okay?"

"Well, I can't promise that. . . . The toys are here for all the kids to use."

"Okay then, I'll mess it up myself."

"Sure, that's something you can do."

"I'll do it myself." She returned all the furniture to the little box in which it was kept and she returned the miniatures to the shelf.

"Will you be here when I come back next time?"

"Yes, I will be."

"And this is your room?"

"Yes, this is my room."

"And the dollhouse will be here too."

"Yes, it will be." Mandy ran out and hugged Lupe warmly. She told her it was time to go home and she waved back at me as she left.

The following sessions Mandy played with the doll-house, remaining preoccupied with the fact there was no roof. She also played in the sand tray, making circles with her fingers and pouring sand in and out of containers. She colored almost every session, and asked a lot of questions about who came and went out of the office, who colored in the books she used, whether crayons would still be there when she returned, whether anyone else used the toys she played with, and whether anyone had ever broken any of them. Her preoccupation with permanence and stability were very clear. She also asked a lot of personal questions about the other children who came to therapy, such as about who their parents were, if they spoke Spanish, where they lived, and why they came to see me. I gave her noncommittal responses such as, "Some of them have two parents, some of them have one parent. . . . Some of them live nearby, some of them more far away; some speak Spanish, some don't; some of them come because they have problems or something's hurting them deep inside. . . ."

Lupe and Muriel reported that things remained the same at home. Mandy continued to behave in the reserved and quiet way that concerned them. She hadn't raised any specific questions or concerns and she was doing fairly well at school, although the teachers had also noticed a change in her usual outgoing demeanor. I asked Lupe and Muriel to come to a session along with Mandy. I wanted to observe Mandy's behavior with her parents.

During the conjoint session, Mandy calmly showed her parents around the playroom, and recounted for them all the different ways that we had played together during our sessions. She reserved the dollhouse for last, and then showed her parents how she furnished the house and how she was able to put everyone to bed at night. Lupe asked about the little friend in the girl's bed, and Mandy said, "That's Daniel, the guardian dog, and he takes care of the little girl." "Good," said Lupe, "he guards his little girl. . . ." "What would happen if Daniel wasn't there?"

"That would be sad," Mandy replied.

"How come?"

"Because she would be lonely."

"Oh, honey. Do you feel lonely at night?"

"Not me. She in the bed."

"Oh, I see."

"Daniel is her guard dog."

"What does he guard her from?"

"Bad things happening."

"Like what?"

"I don't know mommy. Just stuff." Lupe was concerned and looked up at me, wondering how to understand what Mandy was talking about. I decided not to intervene, but rather to observe Lupe and Muriel's ability to tolerate anxiety and deal with Mandy directly. Muriel called Mandy to her and Mandy crawled in her lap. "That little girl is very lucky to have a guard dog," Muriel said. "Yup," said Mandy. "Can we get a doggy?" Muriel braced herself and responded, "Honey you know we can't. We don't own our own house and the owner won't let us get a doggy. You know that." "I know, I know," replied Mandy. Muriel rocked Mandy for a few minutes and then it was time to leave. "I like it when you visit my room," Mandy told her parents. I interjected, "That's good, because I'd like all three of you to come back together next time."

Implementation of the Mutual Story-Telling Technique

I decided to try the Mutual Story-Telling Technique, and asked the family to make up a story with a beginning, middle, and end. They looked at each other and Lupe suggested that someone begin the story. Mandy volunteered:

"Once upon a time, there was a (*long pause*) fish. (*Mandy looks very pleased with herself, and then she frowns.*) Two fish, make that two fish. There was a pretty fish with orange and red colors, and a brown and white fish who was her guard fish. (*Everyone smiles.*)

"The fish liked to swim in their favorite swimming hole. They were jumping in and out of the water, swimming around, having soda juice when they got hungry . . ." (*She looks at Lupe and asks, "Then what?" At that point, the others participate in the story.*)

LUPE: They were the happiest of fish. They liked each other so much and wouldn't go anywhere one without the other.

MURIEL: They felt so lucky to be fish and live in such wonderful and clear water. They played and played all day—

MANDY: But fishermen come to fish. And they had nets and try to catch them—

LUPE: But the guard fish would protect his friend by telling her to hide under the rocks at the bottom of the lake, and not jump out while the fishermen were around.

MANDY: But she wanted to go and see anyway, and her guard fish couldn't keep her from jumping high and looking around—

MURIEL: But the fishermen never caught them and they would eventually get hungry and go home to their own houses and have dinner. The end.

Both Mandy and Lupe looked somewhat perturbed that Muriel had chosen to terminate the story, but neither of them protested, so I asked them all what the name of their story was. Muriel said, "Fishes Forever." Lupe said, "A Fish and Her Protector." And Mandy said, "Sometimes You Can't Always Stay Alive." Her answer elicited great concern in her parents, but I deferred their questions by adding that I would now tell a story of my own:

"Once upon a time there was a fish . . . no make that two. (*Mandy looks at her parents and smiles.*) There was a beautiful colorful fish and her guardian fish, who was brown and white. (*Mandy looks like she is about to speak and I quickly interject.*) Wait now, this is my story. . . . The fish lived in a little pond, and they loved it there. They were very happy jumping around, jumping so high that the fish could look outside and see how people who were not fish lived.

"The fish were very, very happy until the fishermen started fishing and then the guardian, being a very good guardian, would alert the fish not to go outside by jumping, but instead, would tell the fish to hide under the rocks at the bottom of the sea. But the fish was not paying attention to the great danger outside, and was choosing instead to go outside and put himself in danger. The guardian fish would ask the fish, 'Why do you put yourself in danger? You know what will happen if they see you. You will die. Why would you knowingly want to die?'

(*Mandy has started to cry uncontrollably and Muriel and Lupe hug her and comfort her. None of us knows the reason for the tears and the intense response, and all of us wait quietly until she is subdued.*)

"Mandy, I'm the guardian fish, and I'm wondering, what should I tell the fish who puts himself in harm's way. (*Mandy looks up and from her mother's arms responds in a faint voice, 'She shouldn't go to danger . . . she should stay and be with you. . . . Tell her you would miss her very, very much if she left. . . . Tell her to stop. . . . Tell her to stop.'*)

"Well, my story ends with the guardian fish telling the colorful fish over and over to take care of himself, and the guardian fish becomes worried and even tired of trying sometimes, but they stay in their pond, as the fish tries very hard to understand the guardian's worry and promises to take better care of himself."

At this point in the story, I had a clear insight into Mandy's world: She was worried about her parents and she was trying her best to keep them out of harm's way. She had chosen two fish to represent a dilemma about one fish's carefree and dangerous behavior and the other fish's attempt to protect and guard her. Was she talking about protecting her parents? From what? Was there some threat to the family? Was this symbolic of a view that her family was different from other families? Did her family represent the fish living in a pond, who only glance at the world outside the pond? And the world outside was presented as dangerous. But why? I said to Mandy, "Tell me about the guardian. Who is he protecting?" "I can't," she responded.

"What will happen if you say the words?"

"Mommy will be mad." (*Both parents look startled.*)

"Honey, no one will be mad. Go ahead and tell Eliana anything at all."

"My mommy's gonna get sick and die." (*She sighs with relief.*)

"Are either of you sick?"

"No." (*Suddenly, the parents look at each other and they understand.*)

"Honey, are you talking about my smoking?" Muriel asked.

"Yes, mommy."

"Oh, my God."

"What is it?" I asked."

"I smoke. As a matter of fact, I chain smoke. I've been smoking since I was 15, and Lupe and Mandy get very upset about it. We've had lots of fights, but in the last year or so we made a deal to quit talking about it. Well, it's more like arguing—especially when Lupe was pregnant. . . . If anything could have broke us up it was this. We had a number of big brawls about it. Mandy was little though; I never thought she was even aware."

Mandy hugged her mother and told her that at school one of her classmates' mother had died of lung cancer. She also told her that her teacher had talked to all of them about the dangers of smoking. "When I tried to talk to you about it," Mandy continued, "you got mad and yelled at me . . . you told me 'shut up.'"

APPLYING PLAY THERAPY TECHNIQUES

Muriel had tears coming down her cheeks as she realized that Mandy's problems stemmed from her extreme worry over Muriel's health and her inability to speak to her parents about the subject since it was a forbidden topic of discussion. Muriel took Mandy's face in her hands and said, "You've been a good guardian to me and mommy, you hear me . . . a good and caring guardian. And now I promise you that I will quit tomorrow, and I will work very hard to never smoke again." "Not even outside?" Mandy asked. "Not even outside, or hiding, or anything." Lupe kissed Mandy and then all three gave one another a warm hug.

Both of them thanked me profusely and I noted that it was never easy to quit smoking and that Muriel might need some outside help. I told her I was willing to refer her to another counselor who specialized in helping people stop smoking, and she said she would call me for the phone number, which she did. I told Mandy I'd see her next week just by herself. Muriel's promise to quit smoking was difficult to keep and she had many relapses before she made a full recovery from this difficult addiction. Of her own initiative, Lupe told Muriel and Mandy that it was her turn to be the guardian and that Mandy no longer had to serve that function, since "little girls needed to use all their energies just to get bigger and stronger." Lupe and Muriel could not buy a real dog for Mandy but they purchased a life-size brown-and-white dog, who sat on her window ledge.

CONCLUSION

Mandy was a bright and loving child who became acutely frightened and concerned about her mother's smoking when her friend's mother died of lung cancer. Because smoking had become a source of rigorous conflict between Mandy's parents, everyone in the family had chosen to simply avoid the subject by internalizing all their worries and concerns. Mandy's concern for her mother mounted over time and she became distracted by the possibility that she might lose her mother to cancer (a possibility greatly enhanced by her grandfather's death). An educational program in her school further emphasized the hazards of smoking and created an insurmountable fear in Mandy, who began fantasizing about external protectors.

I was interested to observe the interaction between the parents and Mandy, having noticed her preoccupation with themes of permanence and stability. I wondered how the parents would relate to the child individually and as a couple. I hypothesized that something was troubling the child but it was not until I heard her story that the themes of danger and protection became apparent. Neither parent had ever reported concerns over their health or smoking, so I was unaware of the child's very concrete concern until that point. I noticed that when Mandy presented the conflict in her story, Muriel quickly resolved the story, perhaps unconsciously understanding the connection between the metaphor and reality. Finally, while being held, nurtured, and protected by both her parents, Mandy was able to muster up the strength to verbalize her unspoken fear about Muriel's smoking.

Other Story-Telling Techniques

In spite of the popularity of Gardner's Mutual Story-Telling Technique, described in the previous chapter, interest in more general therapeutic story-telling techniques has been modest, despite the documented potential for assisting children to communicate. An early study, conducted in 1936 (Despert & Potter, 1936), concluded that stories could serve as an apt vehicle for verbalizing fantasies. Through them children often reveal their inner drives and conflicts. Despert and Potter argue that primary emotions can be found in stories, including those of anxiety, guilt, wish fulfillment, and aggression. Hence, recurring themes in a story could signal a principal concern or conflict. They also argue that stories are most useful when children determine their own content, and that they can serve as tools in both evaluation and treatment.

Brandell (1984) asserts that most of the techniques utilized in child psychotherapy are designed to elicit fantasies, not necessarily stories. After extensively reviewing the literature, he also found that there are relatively few instances in which story-telling is used systematically and independently of other psychotherapeutic techniques. Some psychoanalytic play therapists may find it harmful to have a child relate a story, since they may feel it interrupts the normal flow of the unconscious. Others might find the technique restrictive in that it relies on children's verbal abilities. Gondor (1957) stresses that clinicians should give children ample room to choose their own preferred method of communicating, which is an important point since no single technique is appropriate for every child. I myself feel that my task as a clinician is to keep opening windows of opportunity.

Robertson and Barford (1970) contend that stories are useful when working with chronically ill children. Kritzberg (1971) developed two therapeutic games, Therapeutic Imaginative Story-Telling Kit (TISKIT) and Tell-A-Story-Kit (TASKIT), to help elicit and process stories told by young clients who may not respond well to a free play situation. Although Kritzberg originally developed his games in collaboration with Richard Gardner, the two gifted clinicians differ in their approaches. Perhaps because of his interest in eliciting responses from children who are "well-defended" and do not use play spontaneously, Kritzberg believes that stories should be stimulus-dependent, utilize rewards, be used as a regular therapeutic maneuver, analyzed according to rigorous categories, and suggest specific clinical responses. He also feels that a story should not include a lesson, and the themes under discussion should not be restricted to the child's story. As we saw in the previous chapter, Gardner's technique is stimulus-independent, represents an adjunctive technique that concludes with a moral or lesson, and utilizes the thematic content presented by the child.

Story-telling is a highly effective technique in getting children to communicate. The uses of story-telling abound: Educators, psychotherapists, hypnotherapists, parents, and others have demonstrated the use of story-telling to educate, inspire, threaten, titillate, frighten, delight, stimulate, and transmit values to children. Children are most often first exposed to stories by their parents, who read them stories in book form. In the last 5 or 6 years, sadly, some of this ritual has been replaced because more and more children hear stories on cassette recorders or watch them on video tapes instead.

Webb (1991) notes that all story-telling, whether it is based on telling, reading, or watching, involves distancing, identification, and projection: "In listening to stories children learn to exercise the power of their imaginations as they envision animal or human characters coping with situations similar in some respect to those in their own everyday lives" (p. 34). Webb cautions that although story-telling techniques may seem deceptively simple, "the therapeutic management and response to the child's revelations depend on a thorough understanding of child development, typical responses of children to stress, and the nature of symbolic communication" (p. 35). She therefore suggests regular supervision for beginning therapists.

Story-telling is used by clinicians as a tool that allows for more free and open communication with children by decreasing their resistance and enhancing their ability to use metaphors to process painful aspects of their life situation. In Chapter 7, we saw that when children were given an opportunity to tell their stories, clinicians could by entering into the world of the story create options that demonstrated healthier and alternative coping strategies to those presented in the story. However, some children are reluctant to offer their own stories—their communication may be constricted and they may literally fear reprisal for telling an "inadequate" story. In some children, spontaneity and joy have disappeared and it is as if they can no longer avail themselves of their natural tendencies (e.g., to play, laugh, move physically, and take risks). Instead, they appear hesitant, uncomfortable, shutdown, and unavailable for story-telling. With such children, clinicians can then move to other uses of stories. Some clinicians use story-telling in combination with doll play. Hoffman and Rogers (1991) describe a technique in which children who had experienced an earthquake were given a "book" with a cover drawn by them on construction paper and stapled pages of stories they had dictated. The therapist can also encourage children to write down their stories in a blank book at home; or mutual storytelling can be conducted using a sentence-completion format (Saravay, 1991). For example, children can be coached to tell stories by beginning them, such as "one day my mom was real happy because . . . ," "Children are almost always afraid of . . . ," etc. Clinicians may also tell children a story that has potential relevance for them. When the clinician chooses the topic and presents the protagonists, the conflicts, and potential resolutions or questions, it is an invitation for children to join in the metaphor.

Brooks (1993) uses a technique called "Creative Characters," in which the therapist selects the major emotional issues confronting the child and develops characters (usually animals) who become involved in situations (elaborated by the child and therapist during the treatment) that reflect the core issues in therapy. Brooks presents this technique at any phase in the treatment, sometimes audiotaping the story (or stories) beforehand and other times audiotaping the story in the children's presence. As they listen to the story, Brooks allows the children to comment, and uses their comments to elaborate on the story. Brooks also may encourage children to draw pictures of the characters, or use "action modality," wherein they act out the stories. Brooks's technique relies heavily on the use of displacement and metaphor, thereby facilitating children's initial communication. He advocates using more or less displacement depending on the situation; for example, he might use names that represent the child's primary issue, such as "Angry Bill Tornado," or represent the therapist, such as "Wise Owl," "Wise Old Person," or even "Detective." The goal of this technique is "to generalize what is learned in the story with its problem-solving strategies to outside real-life situations" (p. 214). Further, Brooks finds that the effectiveness of this technique is predicated on children's ability to use displacement and metaphor to "discuss, struggle with, understand, and master emotional conflicts" (p. 220); children's ability to diffuse and bind "panic-like anxiety" (p. 221); children's motivation to focus and elaborate stories; and children's willingness to become "significant participants" in a safe "problem-solving atmosphere" (p. 222).

Clinicians can be as hesitant or timid about using storytelling as some child clients. During my years spent supervising clinicians, I noted the difficulty for some students in creating a story that communicates through symbols. At the same time, most students eventually became fascinated by the range of communication possibilities inherent in the use of stories. Many clinicians develop their story-telling abilities through practice, while others prefer to use therapeutic stories written by their colleagues (e.g., Gardner, 1972; Mills & Crowley, 1986; Davis, 1990). When developing stories, Barker (quoted in Frey, 1993) suggests that clinicians adhere to the following suggestions:

1. Be prepared with the story before beginning.
2. Vary the pace and style of delivery. Take your time.
3. Give special attention to what needs to be empha-sized, such as key phrases, by slowing the delivery or altering tone or pitch.
4. Tell the story in such a way as to make it interesting.
5. Note the response of the client and modify the deliv-ery accordingly. (p. 233)

Barker also underscores the importance of being succinct and staying aware of nonverbal messages. He states that the use of gestures, facial expressions, laughter, and variations of voice can make the story more vivid, as can the acting out of stories or the use of props. Siegelman (1990) cautions against overly relying on metaphors and the failure to recognize the subtle or implicit messages that clients give.

Kritzberg (1975) states that a story should be action-ori-ented, and have animate or inanimate characters, a plot, and an outcome with a lesson or main idea that promotes the notion that children can master their problems. He proposes three cat-egories of therapist stories: (1) the "mirror" story, which in-volves repeating the child's story with minor changes; (2) the "suggestive–directive" story, which presents themes that en-courage mastery in life situations; and (3) the "indirect–interpre-tive" story, which focuses on a current problem of the child. Kritzberg encourages clinicians to consider psychodynamic is-sues, the kinds of symbols used, how feelings are experienced and understood, and the level of cognitive functioning, in order to more fully understand children's stories and drawings.

Once clinicians tell children a story, continuity can be maintained throughout the therapy through referring to that story. Sometimes, children and/or their families spontaneously bring up metaphors from the story or ask to review it, and at other times clinicians choose to reintroduce the stories. Not all stories capture the imagination of the listener(s). Hence, the clinician may need to tell more than one story until one is found that fully engages the listener(s). In addition, clinicians may want to adapt their stories for children of diverse cultural backgrounds (Costantino, Malgady, & Rogler, 1986).

CASE ILLUSTRATION 1

Sarah was a bright and creative 10-year-old Caucasian, who came to life in the play therapy room: She would draw, tell puppet stories, play games, and earnestly talk about her deepest thoughts, joys, fears, concerns, and worries. She was pseudo-mature at times, but mostly she was a delightful, energetic, and creative child, who was brought to therapy by her concerned and fearful mother.

Sarah was masturbating "excessively" according to her mother, who was quite dismayed by her daughter's behavior. In the first session, which mother attended alone, she described how Sarah was masturbating all the time. When I asked her to describe what she meant by "excessive" and "all the time," she commented that Sarah often masturbated when they took a shower together in the morning, and that she had found Sarah with her pelvis lifted to the bathtub spigot on a number of occasions when Sarah was taking a bath. Lastly, mother mentioned that she had found Sarah masturbating in her bed at night, long after her bedtime.

Mrs. W was a single parent who had become pregnant in her early 40s. The pregnancy was unexpected and she made the decision to have the child only because she had been assured that Sarah's biological father had no interest in participating in childrearing. In fact, Sarah's father had dated Mrs. W only once or twice, and Mrs. W had never seen or heard from him again. Mrs. W had run her own company for 15 years. She had inherited an insurance business from her father and was proud and content to have become its chief executive officer at a fairly young age. She had worked very hard to earn the respect of her 200 employees and to do so she had made an uncompromising time commitment to the business.

When Sarah was an infant and toddler, Mrs. W hired a nanny who became a surrogate mother to the child. When Sarah turned 5, Mrs. W enrolled her in kindergarten and from that day forward she altered her schedule to be home with her daughter every day from 4:30 P.M. on. Mrs. W noted that she had suddenly realized that her little girl was growing up and she wanted to make up for wasted time by spending as much time with her now as she could. Mrs. W's own mother had died when she was 5 years old, and she had been raised by a very caring but distant father with his own workaholic tendencies, as well as a grandmotherly type nanny who had died when Mrs. W was a teenager. Mrs. W reported feeling very saddened when her nanny died, as if she had lost her mother. When her mother died, however, she remembered not shedding a tear at the funeral, following her father's stoic example. Mrs. W did not remember much about her mother and had found only one photograph in which she and her mother were together.

After listening to mother's concerns about Sarah's masturbatory behavior, I asked mother what she thought might explain her daughter's perceived overattentiveness to sexuality. Mother expressed her fear that perhaps Sarah had been sexually abused by someone at her school since she had heard that excessive masturbation was often a sign of sexual abuse. I dispelled this notion straightaway by telling the mother that it's important to evaluate every situation on a case-by-case basis. "Most children," I told her, "enjoy their sexuality even at young ages." She was startled to hear this and added that she believed her daughter was too young to be engaging in this practice. I told the mother I would be happy to assess the situation further.

As mentioned previously, Sarah was quite verbal and outspoken. When I asked her why she thought her mother had brought her to see me, she responded, "She thinks I masturbate too much." Not knowing about the child's amazing use of language at this time, I asked what the word "masturbate" meant. "You know," she replied, "when you touch your clitoris." Wanting to make sure that we were on the same wavelength, I asked what a "clitoris" was. "You're just asking because you think I'm a little kid and don't know, huh?" "Well," I stated, "I want to make sure I know exactly how you're using that word." She smiled and took a professorial posture as she said, "The clitoris is the female penis!"

Once we had the terminology clarified, I asked her what she thought about her masturbating. "Nothing," she said. "I mean it's my body and she can't make me stop." I asked if her mother had attempted to stop her and she affirmed that her mother was "constantly" on her case. "Sometimes I think," Sarah said in a soft voice, "that my mother wants to get inside me and know all my thoughts and feelings. . . . It's like she wants to be me."

When I asked Sarah for more descriptions of her relationship with her mother, she was full of negativity and controlled anger. She described her mother as controlling and intrusive. She said that her mother used to be "normal," but now was impossible and embarrassing. "What does she say or do that's embarrassing to you?" I asked. Sarah responded, "Almost everything. . . . None of my friends' parents are like her."

Sarah announced that she was tired of talking about her mother and wanted instead to draw a picture. She didn't want to draw anything in particular, but she wanted to make a scribble that "grew and grew" in shape and colors. Finally, she created a wonderful free design full of vibrant and alive colors, which looked as if they could jump off the page. She remarked that the time had gone way too fast, and she frowned a little when I told her that next time we would meet together with her mother.

When Sarah and mother arrived, it was as if there was a different child in the room. Sarah's posture and tone of voice were markedly different. She held her head down as she straggled into my office and she plopped herself deep into the couch with hardly a "hello." Throughout this session, I could see that the relationship between mother and daughter was deeply troubled. Mother complained endlessly about Sarah's unwillingness to communicate with her or to go places with her. Apparently Sarah was hiding from her mother in their apartment, and mother was often searching for her daughter, finding her in the attic, in closets, and in the spare bedrooms. Sarah was unpleasant and rude with her mother. When asked questions, she almost growled her responses and I was mystified by the difference in her behavior when alone with me and now with her mother.

Mother was also changed. Instead of the articulate and businesslike woman I had met with in the data-gathering session, she was teary, passive aggressive, and resorted to looking and behaving desperate and helpless. It was clear that both parent and child were unhappy with their relationship with each other. During the end of the visit, Sarah was able to express the crux of the problem: "I've had it with you. You're not me. I'm a different person than you. I don't feel like you do. I don't like all the things that you do. I don't want to be just like you. I'm me. I'm sick and tired of you trying to get inside my head all the time. I won't let you. You can't make me!"

When I asked Sarah's mother what she had just heard Sarah say, she was at a loss: "I have no idea what she's talking about. I spend all the time with her I can. I try to give her everything she wants. I can't understand why she screams and yells. I wish my mother had spent half the time and attention on me that I give to her." I looked at mother and daughter; each had just made an impassioned plea that went unheard.

"Both of you want something new and different from your relationship with each other. What you're doing now isn't working and it's creating a distance that you, Mrs. W, are concerned about. You, Sarah, seem to feel your mom wants to almost be inside you all the time and that concerns you." Both nodded their heads. The session was nearly complete at this point and I reminded them that the following session I would meet with Sarah alone.

I repeated this pattern of a conjoint parent–child session followed by a child session two other times. I was convinced that both mother and daughter were at a crisis point and something needed to change quickly. Unfortunately, the early conjoint sessions proved informative but unproductive. Mother refused to participate in any homework assignments, calling them silly. I commented that there was probably a part of her that wanted to change and a part that didn't want to change. She confided that she would rather be fighting with her daughter than not have any contact at all.

During a session with Sarah, I read her the following story, which was written by Nancy Davis and included in her book *Once Upon a Time . . . Therapeutic Stories to Heal Abused Children* (1990, p. 411).* It is entitled "The Siamese Twins":

"Once upon a time there was a pair of Siamese twins. Although Siamese twins are always identical, these two were not. One twin was very big and the other very small, and yet they were hooked together in ways that meant that they always had to do things together. Because one twin was larger than the other, the larger twin always got his way with the smaller one. When the big twin wanted to watch TV and the little one didn't, they watched TV; and when the big twin wanted to stay very still and sleep, they

---

* Stories from Davis (1990) are reprinted by permission. Copyright 1990 by Nancy Davis.

stayed very still and slept. The big twin was always able to determine which way they were pointing and dragged the little twin around everyplace he wanted him to go.

"The small Siamese twin got very tired of never having his way, but he wasn't sure what to do and he was afraid to speak up. He was so attached to the big Siamese twin that he feared if he spoke up, his big twin would get very angry and hurt him in some way. Even though he didn't like things the way they were, the little twin stayed quiet.

"These twins were such an oddity that doctors came from miles around to observe them and take their picture. One day a very famous doctor arrived and after studying the twins, he announced, 'I have some good news for you. I can separate you from each other and make you into two completely separate individuals.'

"The big twin didn't want that to happen at all, because he enjoyed controlling the little twin and deciding what way they should go. It made him feel strong and powerful. The little twin thought for a moment and even though he wasn't quite sure of how things would be after they were separated, he sure was tired of the old way and he sure was willing to try something new. 'Oh, yes! Yes! Let's do it! Please separate us!' he begged.

"The larger twin continued to insist that he and his twin would not be separated. After listening to the difference in opinions about the separation, the doctors had a big conference and decided that it was not the big twin's right to decide that the little one should be attached to him forever. Against the big twin's will, the doctors separated them into two entirely different people. Once they were apart the little twin was full of joy. He could run and leap as slowly or quickly as he wanted. He could stretch this way and that just as he chose. How wonderfully free he felt. But the big twin was very unhappy. He grumbled and sulked because deep down he was really afraid. How different thing were! If he couldn't boss the little twin, what would he do? How could he be powerful?"

"That's simple," Sarah said. "The big twin could pay attention to his own self and choose to spend his time with things that would make him happy." When I asked, "like what things?" Sarah said, "like spending time with other big twins who had recently been separated from their little twins." Sarah danced around the room, spreading her arms and yelling, "I am free, I am free, I can fly, I can dance, I can go where I want, I am free!"

She asked if I had made up the story about the twins or really read it from a book. She then told me that when she was little she had caught her mom making up a story while she pretended to read it from a book. I told her I had not written the story and that I had read it straight from the book. She asked to read it for herself and when she was finished, she asked me for a copy of the story. We went to the copier as she left the session and she left the office with a grin. That night, she reported later, she put the copy of the story on her mother's pillow with the following written instruction: "READ THIS."

The following session began in a usual fashion with mother complaining about something Sarah had said. Sarah interrupted however, by asking her mother if she had read the story. "Why, yes, I did," said mother, a bit startled at Sarah's direct question. "What did you think about it?" Sarah persisted. "I thought it was sad," mother said. Sarah almost bounced out of her chair: "Sad? Sad? How can it be sad for the little twin to go free?" Mother looked squarely at Sarah and said, "One twin's freedom is another twin's horror." Sarah was beside herself. She yelled, "How can you be so weird? Why can't you think about both the people, not just the bigger one who's in charge?"

Mother suddenly changed her tone and asked Sarah, "Don't you think the little twin would miss being so close to his twin?" Sarah at this point was completely engaged in conversation with her mother: "But mom, just because they are separated doesn't mean they can't see each other anymore. Once the little twin is free he can choose to come see the big twin whenever he wants." "But what if he never wants to see the big twin again?" asked mother. "What if his freedom takes him away for good?" "No, no, no," Sarah insisted, "The little twin will always be connected to his brother because they are family. Even if he travels somewhere, he can carry his brother's memory with him. And, besides, he'll probably want to come see him if enough time goes by so that he gets the chance to miss him. If they're always together, how will they know if they miss each other?" Mother was touched by Sarah's statements. I found Sarah's insight remarkable.

The following session Sarah came in alone. She brought a letter her mother had written her, which said the following: "Dear little twin: I think I understand how I've wanted too much from you and made you feel crowded and pushed. I will try to give you more space in the hopes you'll find your way back to me." Sarah was ecstatic. "She got it! She finally got it!" She then asked if I had any other stories. I wanted to talk to her some more about the note and her reactions to it, but she simply grabbed the book from the shelf. The following story, entitled "The Hungry Porcupine" (Davis, 1990, p. 235), caught her eye and she read it aloud:

"Once upon a time far down in the woods there lived many different kinds of animals. There were raccoons, possums, wildcats and bears, and skunks and porcupines. When spring came and began to turn into summer, each of these types of animals had babies. Now nature generally gives an animal the wisdom to care for its babies in a way that will help them grow in just the right way. But of all things, the porcupine had not been given the wisdom it needed to take care of her babies. So, when the babies were born the porcupine did not understand that she needed to cut the sacs to let the babies out. She just made a lot of noise and even rolled over onto the babies. This was a lucky accident, because the quills of the porcupine stuck the sacs and broke them so that the babies could find a way to get out all by themselves.

"When porcupines are with their children they are supposed to keep their quills flat, but this porcupine mother didn't understand that was her role, and so she left her sharp quills sticking straight out just as if she was ready to do battle with a wild pig. Porcupine quills are very sharp, much like needles, and if you get stuck with one, you'll find that they really hurt. And so when this mother's babies tried to get close to her to get milk, they got stuck by her quills. As the babies grew they had to make a difficult decision: Should they drink milk and get stuck or stay away and be hungry? As you might guess, the babies did not grow as fast as they would have if they had been able to have enough milk. The little porcupines also had sores all over their bodies because they were constantly running into the sharp quills of their mother. They came to believe that was the way all porcupines were raised, and they weren't too happy about being porcupines at all.

"One day, one of the little porcupines wandered out into the woods alone. He was tired of being stuck with porcupine quills and he was tired of being hungry and not being filled. He was angry and hurt and really didn't know in which direction to go. He knew he had to find another way to get milk or he would surely starve to death, or at the very least have a very difficult life. As he was walking, he happened upon a raccoon and her babies, but the raccoon ignored him and so he went on down the path. As he walked deeper into the woods, he came upon a wildcat. This wildcat was a mother who had babies, but this cat understood how to take care of her babies and feed them and nurture them. The little porcupine was very hungry by this time but he was still afraid of the wildcat. He stuck his quills out in anger, thinking he might scare the wildcat into giving him some food. This could have been a very foolish move, but this wildcat was an unusual one indeed.

She had been raised by humans and finally sent back into the wild so that she could live in a natural way. She spoke a language that the porcupine could understand and said to the little animal whose quills were sticking up like spikes, 'You'll never get what you need and want if you keep those porcupine quills out and try to stick those around you.'

"The porcupine wasn't too sure about this, and he forced himself to make the quills even bigger and sharper. He even tried growling at the wildcat, but the wildcat understood what was happening and said once more, 'It is important that you learn who to trust. You'll never get what you want and need as long as those porcupine quills are sticking straight out with those who can help you. You need to lay them flat against your body and trust, and in that way you will get all the nourishment that you need.'

Still the porcupine had doubts. He wasn't too sure that the wildcat wouldn't wait until he relaxed and then attack. Soon, though, he became so hungry and tired that he knew he could wait no longer. He took a chance and laid his quills back against his body, making himself defenseless. The mother wildcat, seeing this, invited him to eat with her cubs and take all the milk that he needed. How good it tasted! The little porcupine drank his fill, and then slept for awhile. As pleasant as it was, the little porcupine worried about the situation. He loved his mother, the porcupine, but he knew that he would never get enough milk if he stayed with her all the time. Unless he kept his quills up with his mother (and got less milk), he understood that she might really hurt him.

"He and the wildcat talked it over and decided that he would come back whenever he needed to and she would feed him and give him everything he needed. And so he spent some of his time with his mother and brothers and sisters and some of the time with the wildcat who understood him and with the wildcat he found love and understanding and nurturing—all the things he needed to grow to be a healthy and well-adjusted porcupine. He had learned something very special from the wildcat: He learned that his sharp quills were very necessary for protection when other animals wanted to hurt him, and it was useful to put them up when he was in danger. But to keep his quills up all the time was only pushing away that which he needed. He learned to understand that he wasn't under attack from everyone and everything, so he could know when it was safe to lay the quills flat on his body so that he could get close to those who would safely nurture him.

"And so the little porcupine grew up and went through life knowing how to handle his quills and knowing how to get what he needed, how to find love, and how to have lots of friends. The other animals often talked about how different the little porcupine was from his family, especially when he purred like a cat."

Sarah reflected on this story for quite a while. I did not interrupt her, but waited for her to process it. She eventually looked up and said, "You know, I put my quills out with my mom a lot. I hardly give her a chance sometimes." "I've noticed that sometimes," I replied. "Why do you think your quills come up so quickly with your mom?" Sarah thought deeply. "I guess because it feels like she's always gonna want something from me . . . usually, and, sometimes, she's gonna be mean to me." When I asked what mom usually wanted, Sarah said, "More!" She went on to explain that her mother was never satisfied and always expected more: "Like last month at my play. I was good in my part, but she wanted to know why I didn't get the lead in the play. She even complained to the teacher and told her I was better suited than the girl who played the lead! She never said anything about my part." Then Sarah changed the subject a bit by declaring, "But my mom has never hit me or anything, and she makes sure I get plenty to eat and that I have nice clothes. She also has hired really nice people to take care of me. One of them was like a second mom to me except she died.

But my mom is pretty good to me. It's just that it's almost like when I started going to school she changed or something and now she's trying so hard to spend every minute with me and know everything about me. That bugs me a lot."

"How would you like things to be Sarah?"

"Regular."

"Regular, how?"

"I'd like her to just be at her job, and I could come home and be by myself. Lots of my friends go home and they are alone until their parents get home. Or, she could just leave me with Mrs. Elliot. She's there anyway, cooking. She doesn't bug me."

"What else would be different?"

"Well, my mom would have her own friends—maybe even a boyfriend. Grace's mom has a boyfriend now and goes out all the time, and Grace says she and her mom get along better now and they do fun things together."

"So your mom would have a life of her own?"

"Yeah, and maybe have a hobby."

"What kind of a hobby?"

"Well, she used to go sailing a lot. She used to like that a lot! And in college she was on the tennis team. There's even a really old racquet in the attic."

"How about between you and her, Sarah, what would be different in your relationship with her?"

"Well . . . if she was doing other stuff, maybe she'd be happier and she would laugh sometimes."

"How would it affect you if she laughed and was happier?"

"Then I think maybe we wouldn't have to be so serious, or arguing . . . if she just wasn't asking questions about me all the time."

"If she wasn't asking questions, what would you like her to do?" Sarah pondered the question. "She could talk about her own self for a change. She could tell me about my dad, how she met him, what he was like. I've never even heard anything about him."

"So you would like your mom to tell you about herself, her thoughts and feelings, instead of focusing on you."

"Yeah, yeah . . . some of them."

"And you would like to hear something about your dad?"

"Yeah, that too." Sarah opened the book in her lap to find the porcupine story again.

"Can I make a copy for my mom?"

"You're welcome to make a copy. Another option is that you could read the story to your mom when she comes in with you next week."

"No, I'd rather give it to her to read." Sarah took the story with her and put it, too, on her mom's pillow. This time mother called for an extra meeting before the regular appointment. She had read the story and had become upset. When she came to the session, she asked if I had told Sarah to give her the story. "No, Mrs. W," I replied, "that was Sarah's idea." "I don't know what to make of it," she said while fighting back tears. "What is she trying to tell me?"

"What do you think she's trying to tell you?"

"Well, mostly I feel that she's trying to tell me that I'm a bad mother."

"How do you understand that?"

"Well, the story is about a porcupine who hurts her young and doesn't know how to take care of them."

"What else is the story about?"

"About how the little porcupine finds someone else to nurture him because he realizes his mother can't."

"And your interpretation?"

"That Sarah is saying she will try to find someone else to depend on."

"Mrs. W, the truth is that this story has many meanings and I can't speak for Sarah, but it's possible that she gave you the story because it meant something important to her."

"Well, I don't know what else it could mean."

"And given what you think it means, what has your reaction been?"

"Well, I just realize that I've been a less than perfect parent. I've also realized that I don't really know how to be a good parent to her because my mother died when I was so young and I felt so lonely most of my childhood."

"And you wanted to make sure Sarah was never as lonely as you were as a child?"

"Oh, yes. That's why I made a point of being home after she got home from school. And that's no easy task because I have to rearrange my schedule so that all appointments and meetings are in the morning or over lunch. It's not easy. But after school was the worse time for me. I hated waiting until my father got home."

"And that's why you ask her all your questions?"

"Yes, no one ever asked me how I felt about anything."

"So not asking would be a sign that you didn't care."

"Absolutely." I empathized with Mrs. W's plight. In an effort to protect her child from the loneliness she had experienced, she made extraordinary efforts to be with her, inquire about her, and accompany her. But in her quest to be attentive, she had become intrusive, and just at the time in Sarah's development when she needed and demanded privacy and was struggling for individuation. Mother and daughter were at odds. The more Sarah wanted to be alone, the more mother approached her out of the fear her child was desolate. And the more mother approached, the more Sarah recoiled. Neither of them was getting her needs met, and it seemed clear that mother had interpreted this story as Sarah's way of rejecting and threatening her.

I could not betray Sarah's confidence by telling Mrs. W that Sarah had mostly focused on the part of the story that involved herself and her negative responses toward mother. I could not reassure her that Sarah had, in fact, been quite clear about how her mother was nonabusive and nurturing, especially when Sarah allowed her to be by not becoming defensive. I continued to talk with Mrs. W about her own childhood and her pain at losing her mother. Amazingly, she told me this was the first time she had shed a tear over her mother's death. This could have been because her father had demanded that all her mother's photos, clothes, and belongings be destroyed immediately. Mrs. W said, "It was as if she had never lived after that."

In the next joint session, I directed Mrs. W to tell Sarah her reaction to the story. As she did, she told her about coming to see me (which made Sarah turn and look at me in disbelief) and the fact that the story had reminded her a lot of her own mother and the grief she had felt when her mother died. She told Sarah that all of her mother's possessions had been destroyed and how, after her mother's death, she was never allowed to mention her name in the house. Sarah looked fascinated by her mother's story. Mrs. W also talked a great deal about her loneliness in childhood, and how no one ever asked how she felt or what she wanted. As she spoke about herself, she often interjected observations about her current behavior. She said, "That's why I think I ask you so much Sarah, because I want to make sure that you're not feeling as blue as I did when I was your age." Once Mrs. W finished telling Sarah her strong reactions to the story, I asked Sarah to tell her mother why she had left this particular story on her pillow. Sarah gazed my way, asking defiantly if she had to talk. She was apparently displeased that her mother and I had met without her knowledge.

After a brief silence Sarah acquiesced and spoke in a soft voice: "Mom, the thing about the porcupine story that I liked was that I was sticking my quills out at you all the time. I don't do this with everybody. I do it with you." Mrs. W could not resist, "But why Sarah? Do you hate me?"

"No mom. It's not that. It's that you push so hard at me. Like you want to get inside me. And I'm just trying to take care of me because I feel you push too hard."

"Tell your mom what you would like to see change between the two of you?"

"Well . . . I want you to have your own stuff to do mom, like hobbies and friends and stuff."

"You want me to do things without you?"

"Well, yeah, but just some things, so you can have a life too. Then you'll be happy."

"And what about you?"

"Well, I want my privacy and my friends and I wanna do things that kids my age do without their parents."

"I don't see how spending less time together will help us get along better."

"Because, mom, I want you to talk to me, tell me stuff about you . . . like when you talked about granddaddy and your mom. I didn't know about that. You never told me. I want to hear about stuff and I want to hear about my dad, who he was, where he is now."

"Really?"

"Yes."

"And will you tell me about you from time to time?"

"Yeah, when there's something to tell."

"In other words, I need to let you go so you can come back."

"Yeah, like the twins."

"So you weren't telling me I was a terrible mother."

"No, I told Eliana last time how you are a good mom; you just try too hard."

"I'm glad to hear that."

"You know, I have the funniest idea that just entered my mind. When you first came to see me it was because you, Mrs. W, thought that Sarah was masturbating too much. I'm wondering what your thoughts are on that subject now." Sarah laughed.

"Why are you laughing, Sarah?" I asked.

"I just did that so you'd stop coming into my room."

"Sarah W!" her mother said in a loud, surprised voice.

"Well, it sort of worked didn't it?" All of us smiled and for the first time since I had begun seeing mother and daughter, they hugged spontaneously and playfully.

Conclusion

Mother and daughter were stifled in their interactions with each other. Mother's attentiveness had taken on an inquisitorial quality, and Sarah perceived her questions as intrusive. Sarah had become well-defended against mother's intrusiveness by erecting a posture of hostility; but the more she fought off her mother's interest and concern, the more adamant the mother became about trying to be close.

Mrs. W's history revealed a childhood of extreme loneliness after her mother died when she was 5 years of age. Mrs. W had never been encouraged or allowed to grieve for her mother's death. Mrs. W's father was a hard-working man, who transferred all of his energies to his work after his wife's death. Although he provided well for his daughter, he was never emotionally available, and Mrs. W longed for her father's attention. Consequently, Mrs. W endured a very lonely childhood, which was void of personal interactions. Though she had a number of housekeepers, they were regularly fired by her demanding father, or in the case of one passed away. Sarah W was a pseudomature, highly intelligent child of 10. She was quite verbal and animated whenever her mother was not around; with her mother she became accusatory, defensive, and unpleasant. Both mother and daughter were highly effective at verbal sparring without resolution. Both had become frustrated with and distant from each other.

The presenting problem was Sarah's masturbation, and yet Sarah reported a passing interest in masturbation. When she described her mother's concern about her masturbation, she commented that her mother was always spying on her. It was later discovered that Sarah masturbated in an effort to keep her mother from invading her privacy. Because I perceived the critical problem to be the mother's overattention to her daughter and Sarah's hostile defensive response, I chose a story from Davis's book that addresses the problem of a "parent, sibling, or friend who attempts to totally control a child and the feeling of powerlessness experienced by the child in challenging the control" (p. 410). This was the story of the Siamese twins. Upon hearing this story, Sarah identified with the smaller twin, who wants his freedom from the bigger twin, who wants to stay fused. Sarah immediately requested a copy of it, which she placed on her mother's pillow. Mother understood the symbolism and made a pledge to give the smaller twin freedom in order that she would choose to return. Although mother made the pledge, her behavior was difficult to change because it was motivated by her own childhood experiences and her own unresolved pain.

When Sarah chose another story to take to her mother (i.e., the porcupine story), mother was flooded with feelings of inadequacy and guilt. These feelings about her own parental inadequacy, in turn, led her to think about her own longing for nurturing parents and the unavailability of both her parents. This story was meaningful on many levels. While mother concentrated on her fear that she had not met her child's needs, Sarah focused on her realization that she was automatically putting out quills to protect herself from mother. She realized that by putting out quills to protect herself, she was also preventing nurturing from coming in.

Mother felt compelled to tell her daughter about her mother's death and the subsequent emotional withdrawal of her father, as well as the fact that she was never allowed to shed a tear for her mother's death. Sarah listened attentively to mother's "story," and they achieved closeness by relating to each other in a new way. Mother was not focused on extracting information from her daughter or controlling her behavior; rather, she focused on her own feelings and experiences. Sarah, in turn, flattened out her quills so she could listen to her mother's story about her childhood.

From this point on, we had joint sessions every time and attempted to repeat the pattern of mother sharing about herself and Sarah listening. In addition, Sarah was able to ask for certain privileges, like having a lock on her door (which she discovered did not need bolting), taking her showers alone, and spending time with her friends, even in sleepovers. As Sarah felt less intrusion from mother, she was able to choose things to confide in her, as well as determine which things she wanted to keep appropriately private. Clearly, the number of positive interactions between Sarah and her mother increased, which created a more secure context for conflict resolution.

Mother became more and more comfortable with letting Sarah go places alone, and even pursued some of her own interests. She found that sailing was no longer enjoyable since she now got ill aboard ships, but found that she could still play tennis fairly well. As a result, she enrolled in some tennis clinics with the goal of eventually looking for tennis matches and meeting new people. Mrs. W also decided to pursue counseling, being interested in the depth of emotions she had uncovered. I referred her to an individual therapist.

The use of therapeutic stories is an often untapped resource, which can be of great assistance in many circumstances. In this particular case, I chose story-telling because both mother and daughter were caught up in verbal battling, and because I thought that I could use metaphors to help convey meaning. Both mother and daughter were very receptive to reading the stories, and finding the symbolism and its application. Both approached the stories looking for and finding the inherent lessons within them.

On occasion, children may appear disinterested in stories. They may do something else as they listen, not connect with the story immediately, or fail to see the relevance between the story and their own situations. Sometimes children take longer to process the story, or they may allow the story to take on meaning on different levels at different times. On occasion, I read the story a couple of times; other times, I send the stories home for children to read again during the week. When children cannot relate at all to the stories, or they seem resistant to listening to "somebody else's" story, I may ask them to tell their own story or listen to one that I make up on the spot. With the following illustration, I developed a tailor-made story for a child who was unresponsive to most of my interventions and seemed to be fearful of talking about her own situation.

CASE ILLUSTRATION 2

Shani, a 4-year-old Asian child, was brought to therapy by her concerned grandmother, who described a painful situation regarding her daughter Lani and granddaughter Shani. She told me how difficult it was for her to seek help outside the family, since it was simply "not done," but confided that she was at her wit's end and felt that her family did not seem able or willing to give her "real" help. She told me that Lani had been a difficult child and an even more problematic adolescent. Grandmother had adopted Lani when her husband was still alive, but he had died when the child was an infant. (Grandmother later confided that she related the stress of adoption to her husband's death and therefore might have been somewhat resentful of Lani when she was a child.) Lani was born out of wedlock to one of grandmother's young cousins, who was not in a position to care for the child. Grandmother had adopted the child so she would be raised within the family and not by a stranger.

She told me that her husband had encouraged her to adopt the child and that she had been reluctant at first. She had not expected to raise Lani by herself and felt extremely overwhelmed by the responsibility, particularly because she was extremely depressed and sad about her husband's death. Grandmother expressed remorse for this situation, feeling that perhaps she had failed Lani from the time she was very young. She speculated that her ambivalent caretaking could be the reason why Lani had been so difficult and angry throughout her young life. Grandmother added that by the time she was in a better emotional position to be a good parent to the child, Lani was very difficult to manage, and prone to engage in temper tantrums and disobedience.

Lani, grandmother claimed, was "a lost case" as far as she could tell, but she saw Shani as a loving and lovely child who seemed to be suffering, which broke grandmother's heart. I asked grandmother to give me more information about her daughter Lani, and she said that Lani didn't wait to be a teenager to become difficult. She wouldn't listen to anything grandmother said from the time she was 6 or 7. She described Lani as "willful and selfish," as often hurting other children, and as doing spiteful things like setting their pet birds free and burning grandmother's clothes. Further, she was suspended from school more times than grandmother could remember, and when she was in high school, she was truant more than she attended school. When she was 14, Lani ran away numerous times and sometimes was gone for months at a time. She shaved her head, wore dirty clothes, and started smoking marijuana when she was 12. There were often empty beer cans under her bed and some of her friends were high-school dropouts and gang members. Grandmother stated that Lani never finished high school, and ran away to marry at 16 years of age. The marriage broke up shortly after Lani got pregnant. Grandmother assumed that Lani smoked marijuana and drank beer throughout her pregnancy. At that time, Lani would often come home and, according to grandmother, "act like she was in a hotel." She would eat and sleep, and then leave in the middle of the night. Grandmother encouraged her to get medical attention during her pregnancy but Lani did not respond to her requests. Lani, at present, seemed to have a variety of boyfriends, but grandmother did not allow her to bring them to her house since one of them had burglarized it.

Grandmother told me she felt guilty because she did not get help for Lani when she was a child. She said that her sisters and cousins discouraged her from seeking psychological help, telling her to pray and spend more time with the child instead. Grandmother did seek help from her church and received some ideas about parenting there. Mostly, she was told that God would not give her more than she could handle. She stated that her religion was helpful in that she eventually stopped blaming herself and put Lani "in God's hands." "Praying and going to church," grandmother stated, "was great for me and my well-being but did nothing for Lani."

Grandmother was very disappointed in her family. She said, "They got to the point that they didn't want to hear from me, always changing the subject, and telling me she was probably just a 'bad seed.'" Grandmother did not know of her grand-daughter's birth until she was 2 weeks old. At that time, Lani came to the house with the infant and for 2 days appeared to be earnestly interested in her small baby. On the third day, Lani left without the child and did not return for about 4 months. Grandmother became the child's "parent," and had had primary responsibility for her ever since that time. Lani dropped in from time to time, bringing the child a present, or "pretending to care" for her. Grandmother had set limits on her "dropping in" because it seemed to upset Shani, who knew this was her mother and seemed to want to spend more time with her. Grandmother described Lani as behaving like a sister to Shani. She noted that when Lani visited sober, she would sit and play with Shani. But when she came over on drugs, she would go to her old room and sleep it off. Shani, she stated, would often get in bed with her mother and stroke her hair, or simply sleep next to her while holding her hand. Grandmother said, "It's as if Shani tries to take care of her mother, rather than the other way around."

When I asked grandmother to tell me about Shani, her face lit up. She described Shani as a sweet, bright, and sensitive child. She said that Lani listened to her and did exactly what Grandmother asked her to do. Her temperament, she said, could not be more different than Lani's—there was never an angry word nor an outburst. If anything, sometimes Shani seemed pensive and sad. Grandmother described Shani as very close to her. "I think she bonded to me, not her mother," she said. "Maybe it's because I was also a different parent to her than to Lani." Grandmother again repeated that she had not been in good shape when Lani was born, and that her being depressed might have interfered with her being a good enough parent to

Lani. She confessed that she found Shani more calm and easier to care for: "Lani would cry night and day; she didn't sleep through the night until she was almost 8 months old. She was always colicky and fussy, spitting up and crying all the time." "Shani, on the other hand, was always quiet, with a cry that was soft." She went on to say, "I hardly ever hear her cry, complain, or ask for anything . . . except when it comes to her mother."

Grandmother shifted to the problem at hand. "The reason I've come to see you is that my heart breaks for this little girl. She has not given up on her mother, like I learned to do. . . . She always asks for her, waits for her, looks for her." Grandmother said that Lani promised the child to visit her more regularly, or to take her to the playground, and she also promised that someday she would get her own house and then Shani could come and live with her. Unfortunately, Shani's mother rarely kept her promises, and Shani was often very disappointed when promises were broken. "Shani seems to worry for her mother," grandmother continued, "wanting her to eat soups, get sleep, and stop smoking." "She seems to be living on the little attention that Lani provides, and my heart breaks to see her cry when her mother pops in and out of the house." When I inquired about the rest of Shani's life, including preschool, friends, hobbies, etc., grandmother stated that Shani stayed close to home and did not seem to like to go out and play with the other children. She went on to say that Shani liked to draw, to listen to stories and music on her cassette recorder, and to watch television. She also liked to help grandmother bake and cook dinner, and she liked to dance, although she tired easily.

The First Session

When I met Shani, I related to grandmother's description of the child, as well as her concerns. Shani was a petite child with a lovely face and smile. She was very polite and soft-spoken. She greeted me and followed me without hesitation. Her grandmother had told her I was a "talking doctor," and she seemed satisfied with the explanation that I talked to lots of children to see how they were feeling. In the playroom she was very interested in the coloring books and began to color happily as I told her a little about the playroom. I didn't ask many questions and watched to see what she did or said on her own. She rarely spoke unless spoken to first and seemed disinterested in most of the toys in the playroom. Shani was completely bilingual, as was her grandmother, and I often asked how certain words were spoken in Chinese. Shani liked to teach me Chinese words and said she often taught her mother because she didn't know too much Chinese. I told Shani that I had worked with just a few Chinese families, and I would learn about being Chinese from her and her grandmother. Again, Shani seemed to enjoy teaching me about her culture.

Early Sessions

The next few sessions followed the same course. She colored in the book happily, oblivious to my presence and unmotivated to interact with me. She seemed very self-absorbed and calm. She never showed me the end product and simply went on to the next page. It appeared to me that she was used to playing quietly by herself: She did not interact with me at all and when I "wondered out loud" about this or that, she did not respond. For example, when I said, "You seem to like to draw quietly," she didn't even look up at me. When I colored a page and showed it to her, she barely glanced at it and seemed annoyed by the interruption. During the third interview, the child seemed less calm than usual. She volunteered that her mother was at home, and she seemed in a hurry to get back to her. I asked her to tell me about her mother and she said, "She's pretty; she sleeps a lot; sometimes she's sick." When I asked her what sickness she had, Shani said, "She smokes and takes drugs, and that makes you sick." Shani seemed worried. I asked, "What's your mom doing at home?" Shani responded, "We have to go soon; she doesn't like to be alone." She remained distracted and agitated during the session, and kept asking how many minutes more until she could leave. Grandmother called me after the session to tell me mother had left by the time Shani had returned home and she had cried herself to sleep while complaining that it was "dumb Eliana's fault" that she didn't get to see her mother. "Don't feel bad," said grandmother. "It would either be your fault or mine, never Lani's."

The following session I asked Shani about her mother's visit and she was calm once again and matter-of-fact as she said, "That's okay, she'll come back soon, on Sunday next." I asked her to draw a picture of her mommy and she tried but eventually gave up. "I can't draw good," she said. I wondered whether this refusal represented an inability to draw, since she had drawn a picture of herself and grandmother without too much trouble, or whether thinking about her mother was too painful. By now I had noticed that Shani had great difficulty in expressing most emotions. She only sporadically spoke, and only to say she was "happy" or "fine." She didn't seem able to talk about disappointment and sadness, or her own or anyone else's anger. When I asked if grandmother ever got angry, she said, "No, when you're angry you clap your hands." That seemed to be a Sesame Street message, but she had interpreted it as an admonition against showing angry feelings. She insisted that grandmother never got mad, and never clapped her hands. Grandmother told me that, in fact, she often got angry and would raise her voice, especially during heated arguments with her sisters. Grandmother described slamming the phone down in the middle of a conversation with her sister, causing Shani to run into her bedroom and curl up on the bed, apparently alarmed by the display of anger. She stated over and over "my ears hurt when you yell."

Shani seemed to be a generally depressed child. What grandmother described as calm behavior, often seemed to me to be withdrawn and compliant behavior. My guess was that the child longed for her mother and, like many children of alcoholic parents, seemed to both worry about Lani and feel anxious about being a caretaker when she visited. In other words, Shani disregarded her own needs in lieu of her mother's needs. She didn't like to make demands, or upset anyone, particularly her mother. Instead, she kept her feelings bottled up, which affected her physically. As grandmother noted, she regularly mentioned that her tummy "hurted" as well as her head. Although she did not complain often, grandmother would recognize that Shani did not feel well through nonverbal communication. Grandmother noted that Shani liked to spend time in bed, like her "sick" mommy. Shani did not respond to my direct questions and volunteered little that would indicate how she felt. She also only used the crayons and coloring books and disregarded the other toys in the playroom. I decided to tell her the following story using three puppets—a mother skunk, a baby bear, and a beaver:

> "Once upon a time (*I say in a hush*), in a far away forest, lived a mother and her little baby girl. I don't remember how old this little baby girl was . . . let's see. . . . (*Shani interjects, "Four years old!"*) Four years old, that's right. The little girl was four years old. (*I have never seen Shani so attentive. . . . She watches my every move carefully.*)
>
> "One day, on a rainy, gloomy day, mother got up, fixed her little girl breakfast, and said: 'Gotta go honey, gotta go.' The little girl quickly said, 'But mommy, where are you going? Don't leave me by myself.' 'By yourself? You know Mrs. Deer will take good care of you. Quit your complaining.' 'But mommy, where are you going?' 'Now, now, you know I have to go work . . . you know mommies have things they have to do. They can't spend all their time with little girls. Mommies have other things to do.' 'But mommy, can I go with you? I'll be a good girl.' 'Now, now, quit your fussing, you know I don't like it when you fuss, I'll be back soon enough.' 'But when, when will you be back mommy?' 'Soon enough, kiss, kiss, bye, bye.'"

(*I take the baby bear and turn it to Shani and quickly speak.*)

THERAPIST (Baby bear): I hate it when my mommy leaves; it makes me feel real sad.

SHANI: I feel that way all the time, too, when my mommy goes away.

THERAPIST (Baby bear): I hate it when my mommy leaves me alone. I want her to take me with her.

SHANI: I feel that way too. (*Sad eyes and frown of concern*)

THERAPIST: What do *you* do when your mommy goes away?

SHANI: I'm just sad—

THERAPIST: I get sad too. . . . (*Long pause*) Why do mommies go away?

SHANI: I don't know, because sometimes they have to work.

THERAPIST (Baby bear): But my mommy doesn't work like other mommies. My mommy doesn't come back for long, long times.

SHANI: Sometimes my mommy is coming Sunday.

THERAPIST (Baby bear): You know what Shani? Sometimes my mommy says she's coming home on Sunday and she doesn't come.

SHANI: Uh, huh. My mommy does too.

THERAPIST (Baby bear): When my mommy doesn't come to see me, I worry about her.

SHANI: I worry. . . . My mommy is sick and she eats junk, my grandma told me.

THERAPIST (Baby bear): I worry who will take care of my mommy when I'm not around.

SHANI: That's okay. God does, grams says so.

THERAPIST (Baby bear): Sometimes I get so sad I get mad too.

SHANI: How come you get mad?

THERAPIST (Baby bear): I get mad at my mom because she tells me she's coming home and then she doesn't—

SHANI: You can clap your hands—

THERAPIST (Baby bear): Do you clap your hands?

SHANI: Yeah.

THERAPIST (Baby bear): Does it make you feel better?

SHANI: Sometimes . . . nope, just sometimes.

THERAPIST (Baby bear): Sometimes when I clap and I don't feel better I get a stumy ache.

SHANI: Then your grams takes care of you, right?

THERAPIST (Baby bear): Not my grams, but Mrs. Deer next door. She gives me soup and reads me stories.

SHANI: When you're sick, people take care of you.

THERAPIST (Baby bear): When my mommy's sick, someone takes care of her. But sometimes I worry 'cause I can't take care of her—

SHANI: My mommy goes to sleep with drugs.

THERAPIST (Baby bear): Does your mommy take drugs?

SHANI: Yeah, and smokes cancer too.

THERAPIST (Baby bear): Us kids sure have to worry about our mommies a lot.

SHANI: Yeah.

THERAPIST (Baby bear): What else do you do when you're worried, or sad?

SHANI: I find my friend—

THERAPIST (Baby bear): I have a friend, and here he comes.

THERAPIST (Mr. Beaver): Hi there. Hi there. I'm glad to see you. Want to come out and play?

THERAPIST (Baby bear): I would come out and play, but I don't feel very good and grams is making me soup.

THERAPIST (Mr. Beaver): Auw, come on, we can go by the park and play. We'll have fun.

THERAPIST (Baby bear): I would come and play, but if I do, my mommy might call and then I wouldn't be home to talk to her.

THERAPIST (Mr. Beaver): Okay then. Too bad. I'll go ask the squirrel to play. Be a party pooper.

THERAPIST (Baby bear): Besides, I have my friend Shani I'm talking to and we're talking about our feelings about our mommies.

THERAPIST (Mr. Beaver): Feelings? Mommies? Oh, boy, I'm going to the park to play.

THERAPIST (Baby bear): (*I turn the bear and face Shani.*) Boy, nobody understands how we have to worry, and take care of our mommies. We can't go play; we have too much on our mind.

SHANI: Yeah. . . . (*Squirming a little in her seat and looking at the ceiling*) It's my time to go—

THERAPIST (Baby bear): It made me feel better to talk to someone who knows just how I feel. I hope to see you again another time—

SHANI: Okay, goodbye.

At this point Shani moved over to the desk and found her markers and coloring book again, and drew with the remaining time left in the session. She had said a lot and felt a lot, and she had been quite engaged in the metaphor of the missing mother bear and the worried and withdrawn child bear.

The next session Shani immediately searched the puppet box to find the baby bear and the mother skunk. By asking me to put the baby bear on my hand, she cued me to talk with her about her mother. In subsequent sessions, she would either ignore the baby bear or she would refer to the bear's sitting alone. There were times when she clearly wanted to address the issues regarding her mother and other times she was reticent to focus on these painful concerns. At times, when I noticed that she seemed troubled or distant, I would wonder out loud about the baby bear and how she might be feeling. Shani would almost always respond by projecting her own feelings onto the bear. For example, once she said, "She's too tired to talk. . . ." Another time she exclaimed, "That little bear has a lot on her brain. . . . You have to ask her some questions." I would also often ask if she and the bear were of like minds about different things, saying, for example, "You and the bear both have times you want to talk and times you want to think," or "You and the bear sure feel the same way about that!" For a while Shani would say "we" when referring to the bear and herself; eventually, she used personal statements more regularly. Grandmother joined us and Shani shared her story. Grandmother used the nickname "little bear" with Shani, who spoke more freely about her feelings. Her somatic complaints decreased.

I instructed grandmother to avoid rewarding Shani's "sick" behavior, since it appeared that she was using her symptoms to gain attention in the same way that her mother did. I told grandmother to come into her room and, instead of making her soup or giving her medicine, converse with and pay attention to her. When grandmother asked what she should talk about, I told her to tell Shani what she did or said when she felt sad, worried, or mad. "Tell her about yourself as a child, or relate a recent situation, just talk to her. . . . After you finish simply say, 'Sometimes it makes me feel better to talk to someone who really understands.'"

Shani made some improvements in her general disposition and I encouraged grandmother to take Shani to different activities at which she could meet children her own age. Grandmother had not pursued any activities previous to this point because she was concerned that Shani would not go. Grandmother also bought an answering machine so that if Lani called she could leave a message. Grandmother stated that Shani ran to the machine whenever they entered the house after an excursion and remarked, "She didn't call again" when mother had not left a message.

I asked grandmother to ask Lani to contact me the next time she visited the home. I wanted to get a better picture of Lani's commitment to the child and how she viewed their future. Lani was unresponsive to this request and according to grandmother, stopped by less and less frequently, in part, as a response to grandmother's newly imposed "rules" about calling ahead and keeping promises to Shani. Within the next year, grandmother asked for legal custody of the child and Lani began to disappear for years at a time. I continued to see Shani off and on for 3 more years. She continued to have feelings of longing for her mother, but with time she adjusted to her mother's absence and her grandmother's continuous care. I purchased a duplicate baby bear for Shani so she could keep it with her at home. Grandmother reported that Shani often slept with the bear and, on occasion, had long conversations with it. The story of the mother and baby bear was the bridge to helping Shani express her thoughts and feelings about her absent mother, and eventually her absent father. Grandmother sends school pictures of Shani each year, and she reports Shani's progress and continued adjustment to life with a vulnerable and inconsistent mother. Lani has been in and out of drug treatment programs with little success.

Conclusion

Shani was a depressed and sad child who had to cope with parental abandonment and maternal alcoholism. Because mother maintained sporadic contact with Shani, she could not adjust to the abandonment, but developed strong feelings of yearning for contact with her mother. Mother was often inebriated, which elicited her child's caretaking and concern. When sober, she often played with Shani as if she was her peer. Shani would leave the house infrequently out of the fear that she would miss one of mother's calls or visits and had therefore not developed any friendships with children her own age. Grandmother allowed Shani to spend most of her time indoors, watching television, listening to music, or laying "sick" in bed, like her mother. When she was sick, grandmother nursed her, just as Shani nursed her sick mother when she was home. Through this reenactment of her mother's "ill" behavior, Shani kept herself emotionally close to her mother and perhaps allowed herself to accept the nurturing from her grandmother that she couldn't accept when she was healthy.

Grandmother was receptive to interventions that included talking to Shani about her own emotions when Shani was "sick". Grandmother talked to her instead of making her soup and singing her to sleep. In addition, grandmother set rules on Lani's comings and goings and bought an answering machine so that Shani could participate in peer activities without worrying about missing her mother's calls. Grandmother found activities for Shani at a local park and recreation area and, with time, Shani began to enjoy herself a little more.

I decided to tell this child a story (eventually shared with grandmother) that included the theme of maternal abandonment so that she could face her real-life situation vis-à-vis a metaphor. Shani was immediately responsive to a story that involved puppets, in spite of the fact that she had never chosen to play with the puppets before, and in future sessions only played with those puppets that had been selected for the story. Shani engaged in a meaningful conversation with the small bear I held in my hand. The story focused on the feelings the bear shared with Shani when the bear's mother left her to "go to work." It is interesting to note that I unconsciously chose a mother skunk instead of a mother bear. This probably reflected the anger I had developed at mother for being so careless with the child. Shani never commented on the difference between the mother skunk and the baby bear. It was too late for me to change the metaphor once I noticed it so it had to stay. Interestingly enough, much later in the treatment, when Shani was going to act out a conversation between herself (a little girl puppet) and grandmother, she chose a mother bear to be grandmother. Perhaps this signified her loyalty shift from mother to grandmother and a deeper bonding with grandmother.

E·I·G·H·T

Additional Play Techniques

THE TYPICAL DAY INTERVIEW

The "Typical Day Interview" is a technique that I began using about 10 years ago, which I found to be extremely useful in the data-gathering stages of therapy with children and families. I use it primarily as an assessment tool, although I have also used it as a springboard for clinical interventions. I have used this interview technique with children under 12, and when I have tried it with adolescents I often have done a verbal interview without the dolls and dollhouse that are normally involved. The Typical Day Interview consists of walking children through an average day in their lives. By using a dollhouse and small figurines that represent adults and children, children can reconstruct their daily experiences.

I begin by asking children to pick a day of the week or weekend. (If children pick a weekend day, it is important to eventually review a school day and vice versa). Once a day is chosen, the clinician instructs the children to select figurines that represent the people who live with them in their houses. (I prefer not to say "people in your family," because children who follow this instruction to the letter might leave out borders or others who might be residing with the family.) Once figurines are chosen, the clinician tells the children that it is morning time and people are about to wake up, hence they should place the figurines where they usually reside during the morning hours. By doing this, they demonstrate the sleeping arrangements of household members. Most of the time you get actual arrangements; however, sometimes, young children place figurines in the positions they would like them to be in rather than in the actual positions. For example, a child whose parents had recently separated might put both parents in bed together when in actuality his/her parents were living separately at the time of the interview.

When children have finished placing the figurines where they belong in the morning time, the clinician asks them to show how people know to wake up in the morning. Children can make sounds like an alarm clock, or they can simply lift one figurine up and start movement. The parent figurines might come in to wake up the children, figurines and so on. Children will give a range of detail. The clinician will then cue children to continue with their typical day by asking, "What happens next?" or "And then what happens?" As children hear the cue, they move the figurines through their daily routines: Parents may go to work or stay at home; children may go to school or to babysitters; some figurines may stay at home with the flu or run errands during the day, etc.

Eventually, children who are interviewed will show their figurine going to school. At that point, clinicians should continue to ask, "What happens next?" and allow children to describe their routines throughout their school day. In my experience, children will go through a typical school day fairly quickly and then be ready to leave school. The clinician again cues the children to describe what happens when they leave school, such as asking them how they get home and what they do when they get home.

One 10-year-old Caucasian child who had described everything in his home as "fine," reported that when he went home he watched television. When I inquired what he watched on television after school, he listed about 12 shows, ending with David Letterman. Since I knew that the Letterman show came on very late, I asked a few more questions. Although this child's

Typical Day Interview started with his parents being there in the morning and getting up and going "out" as he left for school, there was no sign of the parents when the child came home from school or the following mornings. I asked the following questions and learned more about this child's situation:

"What happens after you watch Letterman?"

"I go to sleep."

"Who's at home when you go to sleep?"

"No one."

"Where are your mom or dad when you go to sleep?"

"I don't know."

"They were there in the morning . . ."

"Yeah . . ."

"Then they went out . . ."

"Yeah . . ."

"Where did they go?"

"Out . . . I don't know . . ."

"Do they go to work?"

"Maybe . . . sometimes . . . I don't know."

"What happens when you're watching television and you get hungry?"

"I go eat something."

"What do you eat when you're hungry?"

"Whatever is in the fridge. Peanut butter and jelly sometimes."

"Do you like peanut butter and jelly?"

"Uh-huh."

"How do you know it's time to get up the next morning?"

"The light wakes me up."

"Who's there when you wake up the next morning?"

"Nobody."

"What do you do?"

"I get ready to go to school . . ."

"What happens if you need help?"

"I don't."

"Ever?"

"Nope. I take care of myself until they get back home."

"How long are they gone?"

"Two days or three."

"And who is with you when they are gone?"

"Nobody . . . but I'm fine. There's a neighbor lady down the hall . . . I can ask her for stuff . . ."

"What kind of stuff do you ask for?"

"Sometimes I get hungry."

"So you ask her for food?"

"Sometimes . . . not all the time . . ."

"What's her name?"

"Mrs. Jackson."

During this interview it became clear that the child was left unattended for long periods of time. Although he claimed that he was alright and could take care of himself, I made a report to child protective services concerning possible neglect charges. Child protective services interviewed the child, Mrs. Jackson, and other neighbors, and discovered that the child's mother was not living consistently with the child's father, had a number of different companions, and appeared inebriated most of the time. The neighbors alleged that when the father was living there, it was customary for the parents to go on bar-hopping drinking binges in which they would stay away from the house 3 to 4 days at a time. During those episodes, the 10-year-old stayed at home unattended, fended for himself, and, in spite of his bravado, coped with varying amounts of anxiety and fear about being alone. Child protective services workers discovered that they had prior reports from concerned school teachers, who noticed that the child slept during classes and looked for food in trash cans. Since this child was unattended at the time I made the report, he was taken into custody. His parents did not emerge until a week later to discover that their child had been placed in a foster home and had been made a dependent of the court.

The following additional questions should be asked during a Typical Day Interview:

1. *Television watching*: I have found it useful to ask about television watching habits. In some families television is used as a sedative of sorts so that little parental guidance is needed. Children may be watching inappropriate television programs, which contain themes of violence and/or sexuality. Although there is no clear understanding about how inappropriate television shows may influence young children, I have interviewed a number of them who exhibit precocious sexual behaviors, and who engage in unsupervised television watching. Hence, it is very likely these shows contribute to their sexual acting out. In some cases of sexual abuse, parents may inappropriately touch their children while they are cuddled together watching television. Children are often very intent when watching television and thus may be unaware of the escalation of inappropriate touching. (This in no way is meant to condemn appropriate physical affection between parent and child, which is a desirable form of nurturance.)

2. *Eating habits*: I always ask about eating habits in families. In some families older children fend for themselves, while in others older siblings cook for younger siblings. In some families sharing meals is not a habit, which may not in and of itself be problematic. For example, in some families in which parents have inconsistent work schedules, family members may eat at different times. Some parents are uninformed about nutrition and may need assistance in attending to the nutritional needs of their children.

3. *Sleeping habits*: I also ask children about what happens in their house after everyone goes to sleep. This is an interesting question, which can sometimes yield interesting responses. One child responded, "That's when my dad comes to my bed and does yukky things to me." This statement was not conclusive of sexual abuse, but alerted me to conduct a more comprehensive interview to clarify the child's meaning. In this particular case, the child was referring to a recent episode in which she developed a high fever and her father had inserted a rectal thermometer in the middle of the night.

But the child's statement could have also referred to possible sexual abuse.

4. *Hygiene*: I ask children to tell me what happens in their house when someone is dirty. I ask, "How do people get clean?" "Who cleans who?" There are two reasons for these questions. In cases of neglect, children are often not informed about physical hygiene and may be so dirty and unkempt that other children shun them. In addition, I have seen several cases of child sexual abuse in which what initially appeared to be normal and expectable parental hygiene practices, when evaluated further, turned out to be cases of sexual abuse.

One 14-year-old Mexican boy was brought in to see me by his mother, at the prodding of a concerned paternal grandmother. Mother described the boy as "sullen and uninvolved with peers." She and grandmother were concerned that the boy seemed antisocial and depressed. I did a comprehensive assessment, which involved taking down the boy's developmental history as well as academic information about him. For all intents and purposes, the boy had adjusted fairly well to his father's trips away (father was a salesman) and had an adequate relationship with his mother and grandmother. He told me he preferred to keep to himself and that he didn't have much in common with kids his own age. I knew something was troubling this young man but couldn't quite locate the source of his concern. I began asking some of the questions previously listed, and the following exchange occurred when I inquired about hygiene:

"What happens in your house when people are dirty?"

"What do you mean, weird?"

"No, I mean dirty, you know, like they are physically dirty?"

"You mean my mom?"

"Sure, how about your mom?"

"She takes a shower every morning.

"How about you?

"Did she tell you about it already?

"No. About what?

"Never mind.

"Okay. Where were we? Oh, yes. How about you and showers?"

"I take one almost every day?"

"Before school or after school?"

"Before." (*The boy is visibly uncomfortable at this point.*)

"Do you take a shower before or after your mom?"

"Sort of."

"Excuse me?"

"Well, sometimes, sort of . . . together."

"So you and your mom take a shower together?"

"Yeap . . . weird, huh?"

"It's unusual for a kid your age."

"I told her that once and she laughed at me."

"What would you like to do?"

"Have my own room, and have a lock on my room, and have a lock in my bathroom, and keep my clothes in my own room . . ."

"Where do you sleep now?"

"In my mom's room."

"Where does your mom sleep?"

"In her bed, next to mine."

"And what would you like?"

"I want my own bed and my own room."

"Do you live in a small house?"

"No . . . but my mom's scared to sleep alone when dad's not home."

"Oh, so you have your own room."

"Yeah, but I hardly ever can be there by myself."

"Have you told your mom how you feel?"

"I try . . ."

"I think it's worth us talking about together. By the way, what's it like to take a shower with your mom?"

"I hate it."

"What do you hate about it?"

"She makes me take my underwear off."

"You wear your underwear in the shower?"

"Yeah, until she says she has to clean me."

"How does she clean you?"

"She uses the washcloth on my, you know, and then in my butt."

"What would you like to have happen?"

"I think I should be able to wash my own dick . . . excuse me."

"Does she touch your penis or butt any other times?"

"Oh, no . . . she's weird, but not that weird. . . ."

"Well, I agree that at 14 you should be able to wash your own penis. I'd like to have your mom come in now and we can talk to her about this together, okay?"

"Okay, but she won't listen. (*He calls her name.*) Be sure you tell her you asked me; I didn't bring it up."

"No problem." This adolescent was in an awkward and inappropriate situation with a parent who did not recognize how she was violating his boundaries by insisting on treating him like a young child. Further, he was not able to discuss what was happening until he was asked a specific question about hygiene.

5. *Anger*: To assess for both physical abuse and/or whether children are witnessing violence, I ask children what specific people in their families do or say when they are angry. It is very important to ask for behavioral descriptions that allow children to give explicit information. At the same time, when the child responds, it's important to make sure the message is received accurately. One 8-year-old gave me quite a fright when he responded to my question "What does your dad say or do when he's angry?" with "He gets just like the Incredible Hulk." The Incredible Hulk was a television character prone to violent outbursts. When the child referred to the Incredible Hulk, I mistakenly assumed he meant his dad was violent. When I asked the child what his father said or did that was like the Incredible Hulk, he responded, "He has holes in his shirts too."

6. *Affection*: I ask children who the "huggiest" or "kissiest" person is in their family? I also ask them, "Who's next?" "Who's next after that?" "What kinds of touches do they know about?" "What kinds of touches/hugs do they like the most/the least?" The hope is that children live in families that are physically affectionate in safe and appropriate ways. Sometimes, this query will elicit information about tickling or wrestling practices that the child likes or dislikes. In addition, when children are sexually abused, they may report being touched in ways they dislike, or may refer to being touched in their private parts. When this occurs, clinicians need to inquire further.

Clinicians who use the typical day interview format for assessment purposes with children can also ask their siblings and/or their parents to take turns reporting their daily activities during family assessment. Clinicians not only learn further about the specifics of each child's daily activities, a great deal of discussion, interaction, and insight can occur as family members listen and learn about each other's daily lives. Children are often quite surprised about or interested in their parents' activities, and parents are likewise interested in their children's perceptions of things like being at home alone, their sibling relationships, doing chores, school activities, and so on.

This interview format can engage the family in a pleasant and informative exchange, causing enhanced understanding regarding each other's experiences and perceptions. By reconstructing daily experiences, and using figurines and a dollhouse, children can play as they provide valuable and necessary information to clinicians. At the same time, this technique allows families to interact together in a nonthreatening way as they reveal themselves to each other.

FEELING CARDS

Over the last few years I have seen a variety of tools emerge that are designed to assist children in the identification of emotions. The "feeling" cards are an example of one of these tools. They consist of drawings of faces that reflect different emotions. The feeling cards can be used in many ways. In one case, I was working with an 8-year-old girl who had conflictual feelings about her father, because he had placed her in foster care temporarily while he resolved some work problems that were interfering with his ability to provide adequate care for her. She had many emotions regarding her father but was only able to express her love for him. She felt that if she acknowledged or expressed her anger, she would be betraying him. When I gave her the cards, I asked her to pick out all those that showed feelings

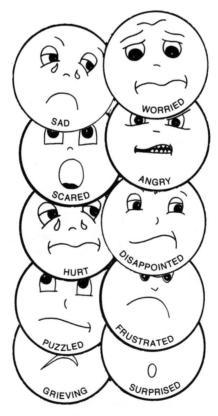

FIGURE 8.1.

she had about her father (see Figure 8.1). When she gave me all the cards, we photocopied them. She lifted the photocopy and said, "I have lots of different feelings about my dad all at the same time." This acknowledgment allowed us to discuss the range of emotions she had regarding her father and her foster care situation.

The feeling cards include a word that describes a feeling. I have one set of cards that includes the words and another set in which the word is covered up so that children can define the emotions they see with their own descriptive terms. This procedure helps the clinician to avoid a situation in which children will not pick a card because they don't understand the word on it, or the word does not express what they are trying to identify, in spite of the fact that the drawing is being selected. In addition, many of the younger children, when they do not know the meanings of the words, may become distracted by asking for definitions that they do not understand.

I introduce the cards to children in many ways. Sometimes I spread the cards on the floor and ask children to pick up the cards that most look like how they feel about a person or situation. I also tell children that they can have lots of feelings at the same time about a given situation or person. Hence, I might ask them to pick up the *cards* that reflect their feelings about a parent or sibling.

The cards are useful in groups and family sessions as well. The cards can be placed face down on the floor, and children can take turns picking up the cards and talking about the last time they had that particular feeling and what they said or did when they had it. Four to six cards can be distributed to each child with the instruction that he/she should turn to his/her neighbor, fan out the cards, and ask the neighbor to select a card, which the neighbor then discusses. When working with families, the cards can be an effective tool to encourage communication about emotions. Because the cards are part of a game that has rules, children tend to follow directions, speak and listen at appointed times, and generally cooperate with the process.

Parents have also found this to be a useful exercise because it can easily be "taken home." When children are frustrated and incommunicative, parents can bring out a set of cards and ask the children to point to the card that represents their current emotions. In this way, parents and children can communicate and use the cards as a buffer when verbal communication is difficult. The card game can diffuse potential arguments, and assist children to release pent-up emotions. In addition to the feeling cards, posters which include an array of faces expressing different emotions are available through many organizations that sell children's therapeutic tools (see Appendix).

THE TALKING, FEELING, DOING GAME

This game, which Richard Gardner developed, is a board game that has the potential to enhance family communication. The game includes cards that alternately ask children (or adults) to talk, discuss their feelings, or follow a directive to take some kind of action. The action cards instruct children (or adults) to stand on one foot and hop, or a number of other humorous activities. Usually, play therapists use this board game on a one-to-one basis with children. However, the game can also be played with family members to encourage information sharing and playfulness. Because it is a game with definite rules, expectations, and goals, it tends to minimize resistance, and thereby give families additional ways to interact. In conclusion, this game is a useful diagnostic and treatment tool.

In addition to the cards provided in the game, I have found it a useful adjunct to ask family members, including children, to make up a few of their own cards to be included in the game, involving questions they think other families or children might find useful or fun. This exercise of creating cards is projective in nature, and often gives the clinician added insight into children and their families.

IDIOSYNCRATIC BELIEF SYSTEMS THROUGH EXPLORATION OF SYMBOLS

Although the effectiveness of art work in children's therapy is discussed elsewhere (see Chapter 5), there are situations in which children's art contains specific symbols that represent idiosyncratic meanings that shape children's acquired belief systems. These symbols may represent magical thinking on the children's part; nevertheless, they become relevant to their behavior. The following example illustrates this point.

Nine-year-old Jeb is a Caucasian child referred to treatment because he had made numerous attempts to have younger children at school orally copulate him. An investigation revealed that Jeb had been sexually abused by his mother's boyfriend and several of the man's adult male friends. The best educated guess of the police officers who investigated the case was that Jeb had been forced to orally copulate these men over a 4-month period. During that time mother's drug habit had gradually increased and she had been prostituting herself in order to purchase crack cocaine. Her boyfriend was supplying mother with drugs and also serving as a pimp. He found that several of his friends were interested not only in mother, but in Jeb as well. Jeb was often home alone with mother's boyfriend and his friends when mother was working the streets. When mother was home, she was incapacitated by her drug use and neglected Jeb gravely.

Jeb sexually abused a child in school shortly after returning from summer vacation. During the 3 summer months, no one was aware of Jeb's plight. When school began, however, teachers noticed an acute change in Jeb's demeanor. The previous school year, Jeb had been compliant and studious, often staying after school to help teachers, to study, or to participate in school activities. After the summer break, he appeared volatile or in a trance. His hygiene was poor, and he had undergone an acute weight loss. Most importantly, Jeb seemed disinterested in school and disoriented. He would often go to the wrong classes or be found wandering around the hallways.

Two younger boys told their teacher that Jeb had isolated them in the bathroom and wanted them to suck his penis. One of the children was visibly shaken as he described being held down as Jeb forced his penis into the child's mouth. Jeb let the child go when someone entered the bathroom. Although Jeb's poor behavior had concerned the teachers who knew him, a report was not made to child protective services until the sexual abuse in the bathroom was brought to someone's attention.

When Jeb was brought in for treatment, he was in a foster home. His foster parent reported that he was very unresponsive, almost detached. Jeb appeared in treatment the same way: His attention span was very short; he would tire easily of most tasks, he didn't speak very much, and when I asked him why he thought he was coming to see me, he said that no one would tell him. In fact, his social worker had told him that he was coming to see me because I worked with children who were sexual with other children. Often, in treatment, Jeb exhibited trancelike behavior, such as staring at the walls. He often rocked in place and preferred to play with Legos, constructing and demolishing various structures. He appeared lost in the playroom and unable to find pleasure in any single activity. He would pick up many toys but spent little time with any particular item, except the Legos. He did not relate to me directly. He would not greet me or say goodbye—it was almost as if he were barely aware of my presence, and often seemed surprised when I asked him a personal question or noticed something he did.

During the fourth session I asked Jeb to draw a picture of himself (see Figure 8.2). I had asked on other occasions and he had always refused. This was one of the most unique self-portraits I had ever seen. Since art work is subjective, I will allow the reader to peruse the drawing and determine his or her own impressions.

I was very interested in the fact that this child's drawing showed a deep blue filling inside a figure's torso. I was also

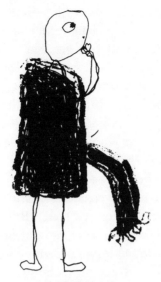

FIGURE 8.2.

intrigued by what looked like an arm coming from the child's body. I inquired about the drawing, and Jeb told me that the "arm" was his penis. When I asked him what the blue filling was in his torso, he initially said, "I don't know," I asked the question three other times in different sessions and eventually he replied, "That's the bad stuff." I responded, "What bad stuff?" He said, "You know," and seemed to withdraw, inviting me to solve the puzzle. I wondered out loud, "Well, I wonder what this bad stuff could be . . . I'm just not sure what it could be. . . ." Finally, I turned to him and said, "I just don't know what the bad stuff is, tell me what the bad stuff is." Jeb looked at me and whispered, "The stuff I swallowed." Suddenly I understood. His records stated that he had orally copulated men numerous times, hence my guess was that he was referring to swallowing semen. "I see," I repeated, "the stuff you swallowed." "Yeah," he went on, "when they stuck their dicks in my mouth." I asked Jeb what that stuff had tasted like. He said it was sour and salty and sometimes he vomited right away, but other times he would "hold his vomit." He looked at me and stated, "I have a lot of bad stuff inside me." I looked at him and asked, "How will you get that bad stuff out of your body?" He seemed embarrassed as he whispered, "I'll give it to somebody else." I realized that Jeb was convinced that he had "badness" stuck inside him and that he thought he could get it out by having other children orally copulate him.

Jeb's picture told the whole story: He had blue filling inside his torso, which was the same blue filling that was inside his penis. I asked Jeb if he had ever seen anything come out of his own penis (i.e., had he ever ejaculated?) and he said "No," with a somewhat worried look on his face. "But sometimes it takes a long time for stuff to come out," he continued. He was unsure but thought if he humped long enough he might ejaculate, and thereby get the bad stuff out of his body.

This was one of the most remarkable challenges I had ever faced. A 9-year-old child was clearly asking me to help him get the bad stuff out of his body. I felt challenged, mystified, and helpless. I sought consultation from two separate child therapists. They both encouraged me to discuss the digestive system with the child, explaining that waste is disposed off naturally through the bodily functions of urination and defecation. I was somewhat resistant to this consultation advice because it seemed like an intellectual response to a child's idiosyncratic belief system. Still, I followed the recommendations and bought a book that described the digestive system to help me explain it to the child. I was prepared to explain bodily functions, with pictures and all. But as soon as I began to talk about digestion, Jeb tuned out and went into trance. A separate attempt elicited the same response.

During this time I talked with both the foster mother and the school teachers, alerting them to the need to constantly supervise Jeb. The school was willing to cooperate. They allowed Jeb bathroom visits only when supervised by an adult, and kept him in full view of yard monitors during recess. Carting her other two foster children with her, the foster mother picked him up after school and monitored his play with other children carefully, being cognizant of his potential to abuse other children. She was extremely patient with Jeb, and although he remained sullen and distant, I felt her attentiveness to him was noticed and appreciated by Jeb. During the treatment, I told Jeb unequivocally that it was not okay to put his penis in anyone's mouth. The first time I said this Jeb responded, "Lots of people do that. . . ." I then asserted, "It was not okay for those men to put their penises in your mouth and it's not okay for you to put your penis in anyone else's mouth." I added, "They were wrong to do that, and they have been arrested by the police and they will be punished . . . it's simply not okay to use your penis to hurt someone else." "They didn't hurt me," Jeb replied, "I didn't care what they did." Jeb's basic defense in his sexual abuse was to deny its impact. "Sometimes when things hurt us, and we can't make them stop, we tell ourselves they don't matter," I stated. He didn't respond. I also told Jeb that I would work very hard to figure out a way to help him get the bad stuff out of his body without using his penis to do so.

I pondered Jeb's dilemma and came to the conclusion that he believed there was bad stuff inside his body and no amount of talk would be likely to dissuade him from that belief. Hence, I decided to enter his belief system and create an appropriate intervention in response. I came into the therapy office enthusiastic and ambivalent about my chances to be of help. I had gone to a grocery store and purchased a roll of blue paper towels. Jeb seemed interested in the roll of paper towels I carried into the playroom. "What's that for?" he asked. I sat down and said I had been thinking about the fact that he believed there was bad stuff inside him and that he wanted to get it out. "I think one of the reasons you've been trying to get other kids to suck your penis is that you think that's the only way to get the bad stuff out of your body." Jeb nodded his head in agreement. "Well, I want to talk to you today about another way to get the bad stuff out of your body. I'd like you to try this to see if you can start getting the bad stuff out of your body." He seemed eager and asked, "What do I do?" I responded, "It's easy; what

I want you to do is to do jumping jacks and then run up and down the stairs and then do some more jumping jacks. Once you're done, I'll show you the rest." He started jumping and then ran up and down the stairway and then exercised some more. I could see beads of perspiration on his forehead. He got tired and sat down on the couch. I then gave him a paper towel from the roll of towels and asked him to put it on his forehead and arms. When he did, the towel absorbed the perspiration, and expanded as it did so.

"You see Jeb," I said, "The bad stuff is coming out of your body." He looked at me and then at the towel. He continued to place the towel flat on his legs and neck and the towel literally became soaked in perspiration. "Wow," he said, "Look at this!" "Lots of bad stuff is coming out." "I can see," I responded. Jeb grabbed the roll of paper towels and asked, "Can I take some of this home?" "Sure you can," I said, and handed him a bunch of paper towels. He left the room with a sense of excitement evident on his face. Unfortunately, I neglected to notify the foster parent about this intervention. It had crossed my mind but I dismissed the idea because I was concerned about confidentiality. I made a mental note to talk to Jeb about sharing information with his foster parent about what we were working on together. As a result, the foster mother spent a week concerned about the child's increased exercise. Jeb had chosen to exercise in his room in private, and the foster parent seemed baffled by his need to be alone and make so much noise.

When the foster mother brought Jeb in the following visit, she instructed him to tell me what he had been doing during the week. Jeb said defiantly, "She knows all about it." When I met with Jeb, he told me about all the stuff that was coming out of his body, but seemed concerned that it sometimes dried up by the next morning. He seemed worried that his efforts were somehow fading away. I reassured him that the important part was that the bad stuff was getting out of his body. At the same time, I could see how concerned he had become about not being able to see the fruit of his labors.

I also talked to Jeb about the possibility of letting his foster mother in on what we were doing. He seemed only slightly interested in doing this but acquiesced. He gave her only the slightest bit of information, and we scheduled an appointment for the following week. As he left, I pondered the wisdom of this intervention, particularly since I suspected that Jeb was making great efforts that I was not sure would succeed in relieving him of his belief about the badness inside him. I also worried about his developing an obsessive compulsive need to exercise, but I decided I would give it a little more time since there was some evidence the intervention was working.

The following session he brought in a clear plastic cup with about a quarter of an inch of liquid at the bottom of the cup. The cup was covered with plastic foil. "Mrs. G and I collected the bad stuff," Jeb said in a loud voice. "Look how much came out!" I looked at the fluid in the cup and confirmed that a great deal of fluid had been gathered. "That was a great idea you had," I said. "No," Jeb said, "Mrs. G thought it up!" When the session was over I met Mrs. G in the waiting room and I complimented her on the idea of wringing out the paper towels and collecting the fluid, and this, in turn, gave me another idea. I then explained this additional intervention to Jeb: "Jeb, I have another idea. I have this special sponge, and other kids have used special sponges to clean up any bad stuff that might still be on their bodies after they've exercised and showered. This special sponge cleans up little tiny particles of bad stuff, so small we can barely see them." I had recently purchased a variety of art therapy materials, including this sponge for clay work. It was a brand new multicolored sponge.

Jeb took the sponge and ran out of the office. I talked briefly to Mrs. G during the week, who said that Jeb seemed so much calmer and talkative since he'd begun exercising. I told her that her idea to collect the fluid had been just right and obviously was helpful to him.

The following week Jeb came in with the same plastic cup. Still with the plastic covering over it, it was almost full to the brim this time. As I suspected, when he showered and dried off with the sponge, he was able to wring it out and get a great deal more fluid into the cup. "Look at this," Jeb said almost before I could close the door to the playroom, "*All* the bad stuff is out of my body!" I restrained my own excitement and stated calmly, "How can you be sure that *all* the bad stuff is out of your body?" Jeb put the cup down, put his hands on his hips, and said, "Because . . . it's my body, and I know!" With that he again asked me to look at how much bad stuff he had collected and after I expressed my wonderment, he eventually moved on to another activity. He took his cup with him when he left and the foster mother told me that he kept the cup in his room for about 2 months and then threw it away. (Interestingly enough, he watered a plant with the remaining fluid.)

Although this was an important intervention in Jeb's treatment, and certainly had a positive impact in decreasing his sexual aggression, he became physically aggressive toward children and adults in the following months. He also became verbally provocative with Mrs. G and elicited a great deal of negative attention from his male teachers and coaches, probably testing his safety with men and possibly expressing the rage of his own victimization with safe male adults. Jeb remained in treatment for the next 2 years with several episodes in which his resistance to treatment seemed to increase and I gave him "breaks." He particularly enjoyed letting Mrs. G know when he was ready to go back to treatment, apparently enjoying the control. The treatment focused on his own victimization, feelings of ambivalence toward his drug-addicted mother, continued adaptation to his foster family, and sincere longing for a father figure. As far as his foster mother, school teachers, and I knew, Jeb did not remolest. As mentioned earlier, however, he did have great difficulty with his aggressive tendencies toward male peers and authority figures. I made the decision to refer Jeb to a group therapy program for young molested boys. The cotherapists were a male and female team, who quickly created a safe and comfortable setting in which Jeb could address his problems with peers and adult males.

Commentary

Jeb was a 9-year-old boy who had experienced severe trauma and helplessness. During episodes of oral copulation, he had been forced to swallow semen; the idiosyncratic meaning he attributed to his abuse was that the semen was trapped inside his body. Desperate to relieve himself of the semen's "badness," he was mimicking his own abuse by orally copulating others in an effort to expel the semen. He had been stopped from forcing other children to orally copulate him because a child in school caught sight of the abuse and told the school authorities. The two children victimized by Jeb were able to confirm that indeed the abuse had taken place.

Jeb presented me with an invitation to help him change by allowing me to see and understand his dilemma. By drawing a self-portrait in which it was clear that his torso was filled up with some kind of substance, he tentatively revealed his belief that the semen he had swallowed was still inside him. The consultations that I sought resulted in the suggestion that I use a cognitive intervention. My attempt to explain the digestive system to Jeb failed sharply, since he dissociated as soon as I began the explanation. It was clear that Jeb had developed an idiosyncratic belief about the abuse, and this belief contributed to his molesting other children.

I proceeded with caution when I decided to offer an intervention that clearly recognized and accepted his belief system. My hope was that if I accepted his belief about the semen in his body, thereby meeting him where he was in his understanding of the abuse, and offered an intervention that addressed his belief, I might have a chance to assist in relieving his desperation. I pondered how to intervene so that the child could see concrete proof that the badness was exiting his body. I thought about using urination and defecation but discarded that idea since the child had been sexually abused and I thought that by focusing on his genitals aspects of the abuse might be recapitulated. Instead, I thought about sweating. The problem became to find a way in which he could measure the sweat emanating from his body. I wasn't as concerned with labeling the sweating as a way in which bad stuff could come out of his body since I thought he would accept this possibility. The idea that he use paper towels to absorb the wetness came to me one evening as I was cleaning up some orange juice that I had spilled on the counter. I also noticed at this time that darker paper towels show the accumulated moisture more clearly.

As I had hoped, Jeb was receptive to my idea and eagerly followed my directives. A problem I did not anticipate was that he would experience disappointment when the sweat on the towels evaporated. The foster mother made a wonderful contribution to the intervention by encouraging Jeb to wring the moisture out of the towels and keep the fluid in a clear plastic cup. To up the ante and, frankly, because I had taken in some of the child's desperation, I offered a second intervention involving the special sponge, which was designed to assist Jeb in measuring greater amounts of fluid in the cup. Shortly thereafter, Jeb announced that all the bad stuff was out of his body and when I asked how he could be sure about that, he said simply that he knew. The interventions had satisfied him. Jeb had addressed his belief system and seemed persuaded that the issue had been resolved.

Getting rid of the "bad" stuff was an important issue in therapy but obviously did not conclude therapy for this child. The compulsion to molest seemed greatly decreased, although the foster mother and school personnel continued to supervise his activities with younger children for at least another 6 months. Although Jeb reported that he no longer thought about putting his penis inside other children's mouths, he began to experience acute intrusive flashbacks of his own abuse, and during these episodes, he would either dissociate or become volatile. Jeb engaged in several scuffles with older, bigger children in school and seemed to put himself in harm's way at times by provoking physical confrontations.

Jeb also addressed intense emotional feelings about his mother and women in general. He greatly distrusted nurturing behaviors or positive attention from women, myself included. His transferential responses toward me, therefore, were complex and demanding. From time to time, he was provocative, aggressive, and openly hostile. Other times, he was receptive, cooperative, and tender. In addition, he was suspicious of adult males and took an offensive posture with them through being openly provocative and demanding. The combination of an absent father and mother's abusive boyfriend and friends had left him wary of adult males. As a result, his therapeutic relationship with his male group cotherapist was the most difficult and the most rewarding. After 1 year of group therapy, Jeb continued to see the male cotherapist alone every other week. The molesting behavior did not resurface as far as anyone knew, and Jeb remained in long-term foster care, developing a trusting and warm relationship with his foster mother.

THE USE OF GAMES

Steven Reid (1993) did an excellent historical review of the use of games throughout history, documenting that many of our present-day childhood games have roots in ancient cultures.

> Games are ubiquitous in modern society and have been throughout history. Archaelogical and cross-cultural studies have found that most recorded cultures developed, or inherited from ancestors, an enormous variety of games. . . .
>
> Many games can be traced to prehistoric times and appear to have had a direct correlation to survival and adaptation. Ball playing is probably the oldest known game. Prehistoric man played throwing games with sticks, bones, and stones. . . .

Tag is another ancient game thought to have been played in prehistoric times. Tag evolved from a spiritual ritual of touching objects made of wood or stone to ward off evil spirits or break spells. This ritual then led to a belief that one could pass on, or contract, evil spirits by touching another human being. Today, the fundamental aspect of tag remains, where one touch from a finger spreads the evil of being "it" from one person to another. . . .

Blindman's Bluff is thought to be derived from ancient rites of human sacrifice in prehistoric religions. The game has a sadistic quality in that one person in a group is blindfolded and victimized by others. (pp. 323–324)

The play therapy literature advocates the use of board games, card games, video games, and recreational games, since games have inherent social qualities in that they require two or more players to interact. As a result, they can elicit interpersonal communication, cooperation, and shared decision making. Reid finds that certain aspects of games can have particular relevance for therapeutic work with children, because they are nonthreatening and familiar to them; provide a medium for establishing rapport; offer important insights into children's personality structures; provide pleasurable experiences; can be experienced as a form of self-nurturing; invite the relaxation of defenses that normally inhibit the expression of feelings; elicit creative energies; allow for the discharging of strong feelings; provide opportunities for the sublimation of instinctual or forbidden urges; reveal unhealthy patterns; provide symbolic reality testing; call upon players to deal with anxiety regarding competition, self-esteem, and so forth; call for the use of intellectual skills; and help children learn to get along with other people.

Reid also notes that the "traditional use of games in therapy has been adjunctive . . . [more specifically] as a tool to reduce resistance, enhance communication, and provide a projective screen for diagnosis and treatment" (p. 340). He notes that the application of games to special problems and settings has increased since the early 1970s. Specific games have been developed for divorce (Epstein, 1986; Berg, 1982, 1986); impulsivity (Swanson, 1986; Kendall & Braswell, 1985); and other problem behaviors and situations. These games are usually played with children alone, but could be adapted to play with family members as well. Schaefer and Reid (1986) note that few clinicians are aware of the therapeutic potential of games for school-aged children and teenagers, although many child therapists have experimented with games with latency-aged children. They note that game playing is currently more widely recognized as a good diagnostic tool, and as able to enhance a child's ego functions and to improve his/her socialization skills. Schaefer and Reid (1986), Schaefer and Cangelosi (1993), and Reid (1993) describe many of the available games. Schaefer and Cangelosi's book (1993) includes chapters on many interesting play therapy techniques, some of which are entitled "The Use of Food in Therapy," "Mud and Clay," "Water Play," "Sandplay," "Block Play," "The Use of the Telephone," and "High-Tech Play Therapy." Although many of these types of play therapy employ a one-on-one format, they can often be adapted to be used with groups or families.

In a provocative and challenging article entitled "Are There Any Rules? Musings of a Peripatetic Sandplayer," Geraldine Spare (1990) discusses the assumed rules that she believes have evolved regarding the use of the sandtray. She lists the following "rules":

1. The sand tray is best used in a one-to-one situation.
2. All the psychic energy and impetus for using the sand tray in the consulting room must come from the client.
3. It is best if the therapist never indulges in parallel play in the sand with the client.
4. The client's sand world may not be interpreted or analyzed with him/her at the time it is made. (pp. 196–197)

She then states that although she wholeheartedly agrees with the thrust of the "prescriptions and proscriptions" listed above, she thinks they should be viewed as *guidelines* not rules (p. 197). The rest of the article is a candid account of circumstances in which Dr. Spare decided to expand on these guidelines. She reports on the positive, neutral, or negative effects of her interventions.

My understanding of her article is that even though we may come to accept certain techniques as more or less effective in certain sequences, or for certain genders or populations, therapists must remain flexible and ready to break with tradition if the situation warrants. This requires therapists to take risks, question customs, and be willing to see each individual and each situation as unique and worthy of unique interventions. Spare concludes by stating: "As with every aspect of clinical practice, meaningful use of sandplay is a function of our own human hearts, and of the ever ongoing interplay between our own centers and the centers, hearts, and needs of those we are privileged to see in psychotherapy" (p. 208).

During the last two decades clinicians have been fortunate to live in a time of professional risk taking, scientific exploration, and a willingness to share ideas. Specific organizations have surfaced promoting the types and applicability of play therapy techniques. Organizations have emerged that specialize in the sale of selected play therapy products (see Appendix). Finally, conferences, workshops, and special educational programs are also available on play therapy issues.

Afterword and Appendix

Afterword

This book is designed to whet your appetite for using play when working with families with young children. It is not inclusive of all possible family techniques. Instead, it is meant to challenge you to explore how to adapt and enhance individual play therapy techniques for use within whole family systems.

I consider working with families and children to be a joint exploratory process in which I am challenged and stimulated and, in turn, do my best to employ creative strategies that challenge and stimulate family members to find new ways of interacting and empathizing with each other. Families can be helped to recognize and use enhanced modes of communicating that don't rely on language alone. Often I have heard adults bemoan the loss of childhood. Working with children affords adults the opportunity to engage in magical thinking, pretend play, role playing, communication through facial expressions, body posturing, and the making of bodily noises once again. Remember being angry and burping loudly to object? Remember wanting to retaliate against a wrongdoer and passing gas to make your "enemy" pay? Remember building fortresses out of turned-over chairs, and using cardboard pieces as shields and sticks as swords?

Play expresses abundantly more than restrictive language. It engages both the conscious and the unconscious mind, the latter of which can relate to metaphors, story-telling, and symbols. Families can process difficult situations and emotions by using play to decrease defenses; consider the following example.

A Chilean parent brought her 4-year-old son to see me because his grandmother had died of a heart attack while she was taking care of him.* He had been gravely traumatized by this event not only because his grandmother had died but also because she had gestured for him to help her when she fell to the floor. When he approached her, she grabbed him and held him so tightly that he could barely breathe. It was while she held him close that she died. The child apparently fainted from fear, or perhaps from lack of oxygen, and when mother came home she found them on the floor together. She revived her son quickly and held him as his whole body shook in fear. The ambulance arrived and took grandmother's body away.

Four-year-old Carlos had refused to speak to anyone about the incident and had had acute anxiety attacks and sleep disturbances. He clung to his mother fiercely and rejected supervision from anyone but her. He would not separate from mother during therapy sessions and was nonverbal and unexplorative, which mother said was uncharacteristic of him. Mother talked to me about what had happened to her mother while she held Carlos in her arms. He pretended to be asleep as she described the incident to me. The first session lasted only 20 minutes because once Carlos awoke he wanted to leave quickly, and mother and I felt that that was the best thing to do.

For the second session, I arranged a dollhouse in the middle of the room and found adult figurines, including a grandmother. I placed the grandmother, mother, and young boy figurines in the living room of the dollhouse. "What time do you usually leave for work?" I asked mother. "At about 8:30," she replied. "Where do you go when you leave your house?" "Well, I'm on leave right now, but usually I go to my work." "Oh, you leave your house and go to work." Mother nodded. "Where did you go on the day your mother died?" I inquired. "I went to work that day also."

---

* These sessions were conducted in Spanish. The author has translated the dialogue.

I handed mother the mother figurine and asked her to show me what she did in the morning to get ready to leave. Mother took the figurine and placed her in a bedroom with the father figurine. Then she placed the "Carlos" figurine in his bedroom, and the grandmother figurine in the bed next to his. The mother figurine got up, took a shower, got dressed, fixed breakfast, read the newspaper, and waited for the others to awaken. Then the grandmother figurine woke up, got dressed, and came downstairs to talk with mother over coffee and sweet rolls. Father followed shortly thereafter, grabbing coffee as he left with the newspaper. Then mother kissed grandmother and went to work. Grandmother worked around the house, cleaning here and there and picked flowers in the garden. When she heard Carlos get up, she made him breakfast and took out a clean set of clothes for him to wear. They then often turned on the television and watched as grandmother had coffee and Carlos ate his breakfast.

Mother looked up, and said, "I don't really know what they did all day." Carlos reluctantly picked up the grandmother doll and took her outside the dollhouse and he rode his bike as she watched. He and grandmother would walk, and sometimes they would go to the store and buy candy and other things for dinner. Carlos climbed back into his mother's lap. I said, "You and grandmother used to do lots of things together." He buried his face in mother's chest and a tear came down his cheek. Mother stroked him saying, "I miss her so much."

The next session mother repeated the play and added that the morning her mother died, she remembered her saying she was feeling tired and might lie down for a nap. Carlos grabbed the grandmother doll and laid her on the bed next to the boy figurine. Then he got up and got dressed, and went quietly downstairs to eat his breakfast. Grandmother slept for a while and then fixed their lunch and took another nap. Carlos watched extra television shows that day and didn't go outside. Grandmother then got out of bed and came downstairs at which point Carlos threw the grandmother figurine brusquely on the floor, more than likely enacting his grandmother's fall. The little boy figurine stood still and finally went over to help grandmother. The grandmother then grabbed him by the neck and didn't let go. Mother said, "Grandmother's heart is hurting and she wants someone to help her." Carlos kept shaking the two dolls together. Mother added, "What should I do?" "How do I help her?" Carlos was very involved in the play. He reenacted the horrible scene over and over, thereby experiencing his helplessness and fear. Suddenly, Carlos let go of the grandmother and child figurines and retrieved the mother figurine. He had her rush into the home and help the grandmother. At that point, he had the mother give grandmother tea and sweet breads while grandmother sat up and then went to her room to knit. Mother and Carlos cried quietly.

Mother took the mother figurine and came over to talk to the boy figurine. "I wish I could have come and saved grandmother. But I didn't know she was sick. And even if I had come home just at that moment, I wouldn't have known what to do, and I couldn't have helped grandmother, and she still would have died. Because her heart was very, very old and very, very tired." Carlos looked up with surprise in his eyes. "You don't know how to help her?" "No," mother reassured him, "No one could have helped grandmother then. Her heart just got too tired and now it's resting." Carlos asked if grandmother was in heaven now. Mother replied that she was in heaven with his grandfather. "Is Grandpa Luis taking care of her now?" "Yes," mother said softly, "He's making her favorite empanadas verdes."

I asked Carlos what grandmother's other favorite foods were and he said, "Pan dulce with sugar on the top." Mother said, "We should take some to her someday." "You mean to the menatery?" "Yes," she replied. Mother called later to tell me that they had gone to the cemetery and laid down several sweet cookies for grandmother to eat. Carlos had insisted on returning to the grave 3 days later, and found that the cookies were no longer there. Convinced that grandmother had eaten the cookies he had baked for her, he felt that he was absolved of any wrongdoing. "She's not mad at me," he had told his mother. "Of course not, Carlitos, why would she be mad?" Carlos responded, "When she held me so tight it hurt me I thought she was mad, but she never ate cookies when she was mad." Mother felt reassured that her son was adapting to his grandmother's death. His clinginess decreased. Mother's sister had moved in to take care of Carlos while his parents worked, and he had spent several days with his aunt caretaker without incident.

The above example again shows the ability of families to communicate through play. Often parents need but slight encouragement to allow them to respond to their children through one of their mediums. Parents have natural tendencies to express through play just as clinicians do.

I greatly value individual therapy with children because I believe that many children need an opportunity to have an experience in which they are respected, given freedom, and encouraged to show themselves and be met with unconditional acceptance. My goal is always to involve family members on some level, whether they are part of the session, or through the use of play. If the goal of therapy is to reunify a family and/or assist family members to interact in a healthier and more rewarding way, family sessions that include young children and employ techniques of play are tremendously helpful and replete with opportunity.

In conclusion, I encourage your creativity and focused attempt to tap into your own innate capacity to play and be joyful. You will set the tone for the family; if you feel comfortable and excited about using play, you will convey that spirit to the family. If you are hesitant, uncomfortable, or embarrassed, you will impact the family likewise. Remember that most families who seek therapy have lost some ability to laugh, enjoy each other, and freely express their secret desires or needs. Playing creates the opportunity for this kind of contact, which inevitably will lead to an increased sense of emotional closeness, open communication, and improved interactions.

Resources for Family Play Therapy

PLAY THERAPY DISTRIBUTORS

Childswork/Childsplay
Center for Applied Psychology
Third Floor
441 N. 5th Street
Edison, NJ 08818

Theraplay Products
P.O. Box 761
Glen Ellen, CA 95442

Toys to Grow On
P.O. Box 17
Long Beach, CA 90801

Creative Therapy Store
Western Psychological Services
12031 Wilshire Blvd.
Los Angeles, CA 90025-1251

Feelings Factory
5089 St. Mary's Street
Raleigh, NC 27605

Kidsrights
P.O. Box 851
Mt. Dora, FL 27605

Uniquity
P.O. Box 6
Galt, CA 95623

ASSOCIATION

Association for Play Therapy
1350 M Street
Fresno, CA 93721

SPECIAL RESOURCES

Play Therapy Bibliography
Center for Play Therapy
University of North Texas
P.O. Box 13857
Denton, TX 76203-3857

Listing of Play Therapy Programs
Center for Play Therapy
University of North Texas
P.O. Box 13857
Denton, TX 76203-3857

References

Ackerman, N. W. (1958). *The psychodynamics of family life*. New York: Basic Books.

Ackerman, N. W. (1967). The emergence of family diagnosis and treatment: A personal view. *Psychotherapy, 4,* 125–129.

Ackerman, N. W. (1970). Child participation in family therapy. *Family Process, 9,* 403–410.

Alger, I., Linn, S., & Beardslee, W. (1985). Puppetry as a therapeutic tool for hospitalized children. *Hospital and Community Psychiatry, 36*(2), 129–130.

Allan, J. (1988). *Inscapes of the child's world: Jungian counseling in schools and clinics.* Dallas, TX: Spring Publications.

Ariel, S. (1992). *Strategic family therapy.* New York: Wiley.

Ariel, S., Carel, C. A., & Tyano, S. (1985). Uses of children's make-believe play in family therapy: Theory and clinical examples. *Journal of Marital and Family Therapy, 11*(1), 47–60.

Axline, V. (1947). *Play therapy.* Cambridge, MA: Houghton Mifflin.

Axline, V. M. (1964). *Dibbs in search of self.* New York: Ballantine.

Axline, V. M. (1969). *Play therapy* (rev. ed.). New York: Ballantine.

Bateson, G., Jackson, D. D., Haley, J., & Weakland, J. H. (1956). Toward a theory of schizophrenia. *Behavioral Science, 1,* 251–264.

Bell, J. E. (1961). *Family group therapy* (Public Health Monograph No. 64). Washington, DC: U.S. Department of Health, Education, and Welfare.

Bell, J. E. (1972). Foreword. In N. W. Ackerman (Ed.), *The Psychodynamics of family life.* New York: Basic Books.

Berg, B. (1982). *The changing family game.* Dayton, OH: Cognitive–Behavioral Resources.

Berg, B. (1986). Cognitive-behavioral intervention for children of divorce. In C. E. Schaefer & S. Reid (Eds.), *Game play: Therapeutic use of childhood games* (pp. 111–138). New York: Wiley.

Blechman, E. A. (1974, July). The family contract game: A tool for teaching interpersonal problem-solving. *Family Coordinator*, 269–281.

Blechman, E. A., Kotanchik, N. L., & Taylor, C. J. (1981). Families and schools together: Early behavioral intervention with high-risk children. *Behavior Therapy, 12,* 308–319.

Bloch, D. A. (1976). Including the children in family therapy. In P. Guerin (Ed.), *Family therapy* (pp. 168–181). New York: Gardner Press.

Bow, J. N. (1993). Overcoming resistance. In C. E. Schaefer, (Ed.), *The therapeutic powers of play* (pp. 17–40). Northvale, NJ: Jason Aronson.

Bradway, K., Signell, K. A., Spare, G. H., Stewart, C. T., Stewart, L. H., & Thompson, C. (1990). *Sandplay studies: Origins, theory, and practice.* Boston, MA: Sigo Press.

Brandell, J. R. (1984). Stories and storytelling in child psychotherapy. *Psychotherapy, 21*(1), 54–62.

Brooks, R. (1993). Creative characters. In C. E. Schaefer & D. M. Cangelosi (Eds.), *Play therapy techniques* (pp. 211–224). New York: Jason Aronson.

Buck, J. N. (1978). The H–T–P technique: A qualitative and quantitative scoring manual. *Journal of Clinical Psychology, 4,* 397–405.

Buck, J. W., & Hammer, E. F. (Eds.). (1969). *Advances in house–tree–person techniques: Variations and applications.* Los Angeles: Western Psychological Services.

Burns, R. C. (1987). *Kinetic house–tree–person drawings (K–H–T–P).* New York: Brunner/Mazel.

Burns, R. C., & Kaufman, S. H. (1970). *Kinetic family drawing (K–F–D) Research and application.* New York: Brunner/Mazel.

Burns, R. C., & Kaufman, S. H. (1972). *Actions, styles and symbols in kinetic family drawings (K–F–D): An interpretive manual.* New York: Brunner/Mazel.

Burt, C. (1921). *Mental and scholastic tests.* London: P.S. King & Son.

Chasin, R., & White, T. B. (1989). The child in family therapy: Guidelines for active engagement across the age span. In L. Combrinck-Graham (Ed.), *Children in family contexts: Perspectives on treatment* (pp. 5–25). New York: Guilford Press.

Chethik, M. (1989). *Techniques of child therapy: Psychodynamic strategies.* New York: Guilford Press.

Claman, L. (1993). The squiggle-drawing game. In C.E. Schaefer & D. M. Cangelosi (Eds.), *Play therapy techniques* (pp. 177–189). Northvale, NJ: Jason Aronson.

Cohen, F. W., & Phelps, R. E. (1985). Incest markers in children's artwork. *Arts in Psychotherapy, 12*, 265–283.

Combrinck-Graham, L. (Ed.). (1989). *Children in family contexts: Perspectives on treatment.* New York: Guilford Press.

Conway, D. F. (1971). *The effects of conjoint family play sessions: A potential preventive mental health procedure for early identified children.* Unpublished doctoral dissertation, Michigan State University, Lansing, Michigan.

Costantino, G., Malgady, R. G., & Rogler, L. H. (1986). Cuento therapy: A culturally sensitive modality for Puerto Rican children. *Journal of Counseling and Clinical Psychology, 54*(5), 639–645.

Davis, N. (1990). *Once upon a time . . . Therapeutic stories to heal abused children* (rev. ed.). Oxon Hill, MD: Psychological Associates of Oxon Hill. (Available from 6178 Oxon Hill Rd., Suite 306, Oxon Hill, MD 20745)

Despert, J. L., & Potter, H. W. (1936). Technical approaches in the study and treatment of emotional problems in childhood. *Psychoanalytic Quarterly, 10*, 619–638.

Di Leo, J. (1970). *Young children and their drawings.* New York: Brunner/Mazel.

Di Leo, J. (1973). *Children's drawings as diagnostic aids.* New York: Brunner/Mazel.

Di Leo, J. (1983). *Interpreting children's drawings.* New York: Brunner/Mazel.

Dowling, E., & Jones, H. (1978). Small children seen and heard in family therapy. *Journal of Child Psychotherapy, 4*, 87–96.

Epstein, Y. M. (1986). Feedback and this could happen: Two therapeutic games for children of divorce. In C. E. Schaefer & S. Reid (Eds.), *Game play: Therapeutic use of childhood games* (pp. 159–186). New York: Wiley.

Erikson, E. H. (1963). *Childhood and society.* New York: W. W. Norton.

Esman, A. H. (1983). Psychoanalytic play therapy. In C. E. Schaefer & K. O'Connor (Eds.), *Handbook of play therapy* (pp. 11–20). New York: Wiley.

Family Puppet Interview. (1981). You can learn a lot from a lobster [videotape]. (Available from University of Pittsburgh, UPIC Library, Pittsburgh, PA)

Fraiberg, S. (1965). A comparison of the analytic method in two stages of child analysis. *Journal of the American Academy of Child Psychiatry, 4,* 387–400.

Frey, D. E. (1993). Learning by metaphor. In C. E. Schaefer (Ed.), *The therapeutic powers of play* (pp. 223–240). Northvale, NJ: Jason Aronson.

Friedrich, W. N. (Ed.). (1991). *Casebook of sexual abuse treatment.* New York: W. W. Norton.

Fries, M. (1937). Play technique in the analysis of young children. *Psychoanalytic Review, 24,* 233–245.

Fulweiler, C. R. (1967). No man's land. In J. Haley & L. Hoffman (Eds.), *Techniques of family therapy.* New York: Basic Books.

Gardner, R. A. (1971). *Therapeutic communication with children: The mutual storytelling technique.* New York: Science House.

Gardner, R. A. (1972). *Dr. Gardner's stories about the real world.* Cresskill, NJ: Creative Therapeutics.

Gardner, R. A. (1993). Mutual storytelling. In C. E. Schaefer & D. M. Cangelosi (Eds.), *Play therapy techniques* (pp.199–211). Northvale, NJ: Jason Aronson.

Gil, E. (1991). *The healing power of play: Working with abused children.* New York: Guilford Press.

Ginott, H. G. (1961). *Group psychotherapy with children.* New York: McGraw-Hill.

Gondor, L. H. (1957). Use of fantasy communications in child psychotherapy. *American Journal of Psychotherapy, 5,* 323–335.

Gravitz, M. A. (1967). Marital status and figure drawing choice in normal adults. *Journal of Projective Techniques and Personal Assessment, 31,* 86–87.

Green, R. J., & Framo, J. L. (Eds.). (1981). *Family therapy: Major contributions.* New York: International Universities Press.

Griff, M. D. (1983). Family play therapy. In C. E. Schaefer & K. J. O'Connor (Eds.), *Handbook of play therapy* (pp. 65–75). New York: Wiley.

Guerney, B. G. Jr. (1964). Filial therapy: Description and rationale. *Journal of Consulting Psychology, 28,* 303–310, 450–460.

Guerney, L. F. (1983). Client centered (non-directive) play therapy. In C. E. Schaefer & K. J. O'Connor (Eds.), *Handbook of play therapy* (pp. 21–64). New York: Wiley.

Guttman, H. A. (1975). The child's participation in conjoint family therapy. *Journal of the American Academy of Child Psychiatry, 14,* 490–499.

Haley, J. (1961). Development of theory: A history of research project. In C. E. Sluzki & D. C. Ransom (Eds.), *Double bind: The foundation of a communicational approach to the family*. New York: Grune & Stratton.

Haley, J., & Hoffman, L. (Eds.). (1967). *Techniques of family therapy*. New York: Basic Books.

Hambidge, G. (1955). Structured play therapy. *American Journal of Orthopsychiatry, 25*, 601–617.

Hammer, E. (1968). *The clinical application of projective drawings*. Springfield, IL: Charles C. Thomas.

Haworth, M. R. (1968). Doll play and puppetry. In A. I. Rain (Ed.), *Projective techniques in personality assessment* (pp. 327–365). New York: Springer.

Haworth, M. R. (1990). *A child's therapy: Hour by hour*. Madison, CT: International Universities Press.

Hoffman, J., & Rogers, P. (1991). A crisis play group in a shelter following the Santa Cruz earthquake. In N. Boyd Webb (Ed.), *Play therapy with children in crisis: A casebook for practitioners* (pp. 379–395), New York: Guilford Press.

Hulse, W. C. (1951). The emotionally disturbed child draws his family. *Quarterly Journal of Child Behavior, 3*, 152–174.

Irwin, E. C. (1993). Using puppets for assessment. In C. E. Schaefer & D. M. Cangelosi (Eds.), *Play therapy techniques* (pp. 69–81). Northvale, NJ: Jason Aronson.

Irwin, E., & Kovacs, A. (1979). Analysis of children's drawings and stories. *Journal of the Association for Care of Children in Hospitals, 8*, 39–45.

Irwin, E. C., & Malloy, E. S. (1975). Family puppet interview. *Family Process, 14*, 170–191.

Irwin, E., Portner, E. S., Elmer, E., & Petti, T. (1981). Joyless children: A study of the effects of abuse of time. In I. Jakab (Ed.), *The personality of the therapist: Proceedings of the 1981 International Congress of the American Society of the Psychopathology of Expression*. Basel, Switzerland: Karger.

Irwin, E., & Shapiro, M. (1975). Puppetry as a diagnostic and therapeutic technique. In I. Jakab (Ed.), *Psychiatry and art* (Vol. 4). Basel, Switzerland: Karger.

Johnson, T. C. (1993). Group therapy. In E. Gil & T. C. Johnson (Eds.), *Sexualized children: Assessment and treatment of sexualized children and children who molest* (pp. 211–275). Rockville, MD: Launch Press.

Jones, S. L. (1980). *Family therapy*. Bowie, MD: Prentice-Hall.

Kalff, D. (1980). *Sandplay*. Boston, MA: Sigo Press.

Kaufman, B., & Wohl, A. (1992). *Casualties of childhood: A developmental perspective on sexual abuse using projective drawings*. New York: Brunner/Mazel.

Keith, D. V., & Whitaker, C. A. (1977). The divorce labyrinth. In P. Papp (Ed.), *Family therapy: Full-length case studies* (pp. 117–133). New York: Gardner.

Keith, D. V., & Whitaker, C. A. (1981). Play therapy: A paradigm for work with families. *Journal of Marital and Family Therapy, 7*, 243–254.

Kelley, S. J. (1984). The use of art therapy with sexually abused children. *Journal of Psychosocial Nursing, 22*, 12–18.

Kellogg, R. (1970). *Analyzing children's art*. Palo Alto, CA: Mayfield.

Kendall, P. C., & Braswell, L. (1985). *Cognitive–behavioral therapy for impulsive children*. New York: Guilford Press.

Klein, M. (1937). *The psychoanalysis of children* (2nd ed.). London: Hogarth Press.

Kobak, R. R., & Waters, D. B. (1984). Family therapy as a rite of passage: Play's the thing. *Family Process, 23*, 89–100.

Korner, S., & Brown, G. (1990). Exclusion of children from family psychotherapy: Family therapists' beliefs and practices. *Journal of Family Psychology, 3*, 420–430.

Kraft, I. A. (1980). Group therapy with children and adolescents. In G. P. Sholevar, R. M. Benson, & B. J. Blinder (Eds.), *Emotional disorders in children and adolescents* (pp. 109–133). New York: Spectrum.

Kramer, E. (1971). *Art as therapy with children*. New York: Schocken Books.

Kritzberg, N. (1971). TASKIT (Tell-a-Story-Kit), the therapeutic story-telling word game. *Acta Paedopsychiatrica, 38*, 231–244.

Kritzberg, N. I. (1975). *The structured therapeutic game method of psychoanalytic psychotherapy*. Hicksville, NY: Exposition.

Kwiatkowska, H. Y. (1967). Family art therapy. *Family Process, 6*(1), 33–57.

Kwiatkowska, H. Y. (1975). Family art therapy: Experiments with a new technique. In E. Ulman & P. Dachinger (Eds.), *Art therapy: In theory and practice* (pp. 113–125). New York: Schocken Books.

Kwiatkowska, H. (1978). *Family therapy and evaluation through art*. Springfield, IL: Charles C. Thomas.

Landgarten, H. B. (1981). *Clinical art therapy: A comprehensive guide*. New York: Brunner/Mazel.

Levy, D. (1938). Release therapy in young children. *Psychiatry, 1*, 387–389.

Levenson, R. L., & Herman, J. (1993). Role playing. In C. E. Schaefer & D. M. Cangelosi (Eds.), *Play therapy techniques* (pp. 225–237). Northvale, NJ: Jason Aronson.

Linesch, D. (Ed.). (1993). *Art therapy with families in crisis: Overcoming resistance through nonverbal expression.* New York: Brunner/Mazel.

Linn, S. (1977). Puppets and hospitalized children: Talking about feelings. *Journal for the Association of the Care of Children in Hospitals, 5,* 5–11.

Machover, K. (1949). *Personality projection in the drawing of the human figure.* Springfield, IL: Charles C. Thomas.

Malchiodi, C. (1990). *Breaking the silence: Art therapy with children from violent homes.* New York: Brunner/Mazel.

Mandell, J. G., Damon, L., Castaldo, P., Tauber, E., Monise, L., & Larsen, N. (1990). *Group treatment for sexually abused children.* New York: Guilford Press.

Martinez, K. J., & Valdez, D. M. (1992). Cultural considerations in play therapy with Hispanic children. In L. A. Vargas & J. D. Koss-Chioino (Eds.), *Working with culture: Psychotherapeutic interventions with ethnic minority children and adolescents* (pp. 85–103). San Francisco, CA: Jossey-Bass.

Mills, J. C., & Crowley, R. J. (1986). *Therapeutic metaphors for children and the child within.* New York: Brunner/Mazel.

Minuchin, S. (1974). *Families and family therapy.* Cambridge, MA: Harvard University Press.

Montalvo, B., & Haley, J. (1973). In defense of child therapy. *Family Process, 12,* 227–244.

Moustakas, C. (1966). *The child's discovery of himself.* New York: Ballantine.

Nagera, H. (1980). Child psychoanalysis. In G. P. Sholevar, R. M. Benton, & B. J. Blinder (Eds.), *Emotional disorder in children and adolescents* (pp. 17–23). New York: Spectrum.

Naumburg, M. (1966). *Dynamically oriented art therapy: Its principles and practice.* New York: Grune & Stratton.

Nickerson, E. T. (1973, Spring). Psychology of play and play therapy in classroom activities. *Educating Children,* 1–6.

Oster, G. D., & Gould, P. (1987). *Using drawings in assessment and therapy.* New York: Brunner/Mazel.

Palazzoli, M. S., Boscolo, L., Cecchin, G., & Prata, G. (1981). *Paradox and counterparadox: A new model in the therapy of the family in schizophrenic transaction.* New York: Jason Aronson.

Piaget, J. (1969). *The mechanisms of perception.* New York: Basic Books.

References

Portner, E. (1981). *A normative study of the spontaneous puppet stories of eight-year-old children.* Unpublished doctoral dissertation, University of Pittsburgh, Pittsburgh.

Reid, S. (1993). Game play. In C. E. Schaefer (Ed.), *The therapeutic powers of play* (323–348). Northvale, NJ: Jason Aronson.

Rhyne, J. (1973). *The gestalt art experience.* Monterey, CA: Brooks/Cole.

Robertson, M., & Barford, F. (1970). Story-making in psychotherapy with a chronically-ill child. *Psychotherapy: Theory, Research and Practice, 7,* 104–107.

Rogers, C. (1951). *Client-centered therapy.* Boston: Houghton- Mifflin.

Rothenberg, L., & Schiffer, M. (1966). The therapeutic play group—a case study. *Exceptional Children, 32,* 483–486.

Rubin, J. A. (1978). *Child art therapy.* New York: Van Nostrand Reinhold.

Safer, D. (1965). Conjoint play therapy for the young child and his parent. *Archives of General Psychiatry, 13,* 320–326.

Sandler, J., Kennedy, H., & Tyson, R. (1980). *The technique of child psychoanalysis.* Cambridge, MA: Harvard University Press.

Saravay, B. (1991). Short-term play therapy with two preschool brothers following sudden parental death. In N. Boyd Webb (Ed.), *Play therapy with children in crisis: A casebook for practitioners* (pp. 177–200). New York: Guilford Press.

Satir, V. (1964). *Conjoint family therapy.* Palo Alto, CA: Science & Behavior Books.

Satir, V. (1972). *Peoplemaking.* Palo Alto, CA: Science & Behavior Books.

Schaefer, C., & Carey, L. (1994). *Family play therapy.* New York: Jason Aronson.

Schaefer, C. E. (1980). Play therapy. In G. P. Sholevar, R. M. Benson, & B. J. Blinder (Eds.), *Emotional disorders in children and adolescents.* New York: Spectrum.

Schaefer, C. E. (Ed.). (1993). *The therapeutic powers of play.* Northvale, NJ: Jason Aronson.

Schaefer, C. E. (1983). Play therapy. In C. E. Schaefer & K. J. O'Connor (Eds.), *Handbook of play therapy* (pp. 95–106). New York: Wiley.

Schaefer, C. E. & Cangelosi, D. M. (Eds.). (1993). *Play therapy techniques.* Northvale, NJ: Jason Aronson.

Schaefer, C. E. & O'Connor, K. J. (1983). *Handbook of play therapy.* New York: Wiley.

Schaefer, C. E., & Reid, S. E. (Eds.). (1986). *Game play: Therapeutic use of childhood games.* New York: Wiley.

Scharff, D. E., & Scharff, J. S. (1987). *Object relations family therapy.* Northvale, NJ: Jason Aronson.

References

Sheedy, B. C. (1978). The creative encounter: Meeting through play in conjoint family therapy. *Dissertation Abstracts International, 38*(8), 3907-B.

Siegelman, E. (1990). *Metaphor and meaning in psychotherapy*. New York: Guilford Press.

Silverman, M., & Silverman, M. (1962, November). Psychiatry inside the family circle. *Saturday Evening Post*, 46–51.

Singer, D. G. (1993). *Playing for their lives: Helping troubled children through play therapy*. New York: Free Press.

Sobol, B. (1982). Art therapy and strategic family therapy. *American Journal of Art Therapy, 21*, 23–31.

Solomon, J. (1938). Active play therapy. *American Journal of Orthopsychiatry, 8*, 479–498.

Sours, J. A. (1980). Preschool-age children. In G. P. Sholevar, R. M. Benson, & B. J. Blinder (Eds.), *Emotional disorders in children and adolescents* (pp. 271–282). New York: Spectrum.

Spare, G. H. (1990). Are there any rules? Musings of a peripatetic sandplayer. In K. Bradway, K. A. Signell, G. H. Spare, C. T. Stewart, L. H. Stewart, & C. Thompson (Eds.), *Sandplay studies: Origins of theory and practice* (pp. 195–208). Boston, MA: Sigo Press.

Swanson, A. J. (1986). Using games to improve self-control deficits in children. In C. E. Schaefer & S. E. Reid (Eds.), *Game play: The therapeutic uses of childhood games* (pp. 233–243). New York: Wiley.

Ulman, E. (1975). Art therapy: Problems of definition. In E. Ulman & P. Dachinger (Eds.), *Art therapy: In theory and practice* (pp. 3–13). New York: Schocken Books.

Ulman, E., & Dachinger, P. (Eds.). (1975). *Art therapy: In theory and practice*. New York: Schocken Books.

Villeneuve, C. (1979). The specific participation of the child in family therapy. *Journal of the American Academy of Child Psychiatry, 18*(1), 44–53.

Von Neuman, J., & Morgenstern, O. (1947). *Theory of games and economic behavior*. Princeton, NJ: Princeton University Press.

Webb, N. B. (Ed.). (1991). *Playing for their lives: Helping troubled children through play therapy*. New York: Free Press.

White, R. W. (1966). *Lives in progress* (2nd ed.). New York: Holt, Rinehart & Winston.

White, M., & Epston, D. (1990). *Narrative means to therapeutic ends*. New York: W. W. Norton.

Winnicott, D. W. (1971). *Therapeutic consultations in child psychiatry*. New York: Basic Books.

References

Wohl, A., & Kaufman, B. (1985). *Silent screams and hidden cries: An interpretation of artwork by children from violent homes.* New York: Brunner/Mazel.

Woltmann, A. G. (1940). The use of puppetry in understanding children. *Mental Hygiene, 24,* 445–458.

Yalom, I. D. (1975). *The theory and practice of group psychotherapy* (2nd ed.). New York: Basic Books.

Zilbach, J. J. (1986). *Young children in family therapy.* New York: Brunner/Mazel.

Zilbach, J. J., Bergel, E., & Gass, C. (1972). Role of the young child in family therapy. In C. J. Sager & H. S. Kaplan (Eds.), *Progress in group and family therapy* (pp. 385–399). New York: Brunner/Mazel.

Index